Pain: A Very Short Introduction

VERY SHORT INTRODUCTIONS are for anyone wanting a stimulating and accessible way into a new subject. They are written by experts, and have been translated into more than 45 different languages.

The series began in 1995, and now covers a wide variety of topics in every discipline. The VSI library now contains over 500 volumes—a Very Short Introduction to everything from Psychology and Philosophy of Science to American History and Relativity—and continues to grow in every subject area.

Very Short Introductions available now:

ACCOUNTING Christopher Nobes
ADOLESCENCE Peter K. Smith
ADVERTISING Winston Fletcher
AFRICAN AMERICAN RELIGION
    Eddie S. Glaude Jr
AFRICAN HISTORY
    John Parker and Richard Rathbone
AFRICAN RELIGIONS
    Jacob K. Olupona
AGEING Nancy A. Pachana
AGNOSTICISM Robin Le Poidevin
AGRICULTURE Paul Brassley and
    Richard Soffe
ALEXANDER THE GREAT
    Hugh Bowden
ALGEBRA Peter M. Higgins
AMERICAN HISTORY Paul S. Boyer
AMERICAN IMMIGRATION
    David A. Gerber
AMERICAN LEGAL HISTORY
    G. Edward White
AMERICAN POLITICAL HISTORY
    Donald Critchlow
AMERICAN POLITICAL PARTIES
    AND ELECTIONS L. Sandy Maisel
AMERICAN POLITICS
    Richard M. Valelly
THE AMERICAN PRESIDENCY
    Charles O. Jones
THE AMERICAN REVOLUTION
    Robert J. Allison
AMERICAN SLAVERY
    Heather Andrea Williams
THE AMERICAN WEST Stephen Aron

AMERICAN WOMEN'S HISTORY
    Susan Ware
ANAESTHESIA Aidan O'Donnell
ANARCHISM Colin Ward
ANCIENT ASSYRIA Karen Radner
ANCIENT EGYPT Ian Shaw
ANCIENT EGYPTIAN ART AND
    ARCHITECTURE Christina Riggs
ANCIENT GREECE Paul Cartledge
THE ANCIENT NEAR EAST
    Amanda H. Podany
ANCIENT PHILOSOPHY Julia Annas
ANCIENT WARFARE
    Harry Sidebottom
ANGELS David Albert Jones
ANGLICANISM Mark Chapman
THE ANGLO-SAXON AGE John Blair
ANIMAL BEHAVIOUR
    Tristram D. Wyatt
THE ANIMAL KINGDOM
    Peter Holland
ANIMAL RIGHTS David DeGrazia
THE ANTARCTIC Klaus Dodds
ANTISEMITISM Steven Beller
ANXIETY Daniel Freeman and
    Jason Freeman
THE APOCRYPHAL GOSPELS
    Paul Foster
ARCHAEOLOGY Paul Bahn
ARCHITECTURE Andrew Ballantyne
ARISTOCRACY William Doyle
ARISTOTLE Jonathan Barnes
ART HISTORY Dana Arnold
ART THEORY Cynthia Freeland

ASIAN AMERICAN HISTORY
    Madeline Y. Hsu
ASTROBIOLOGY David C. Catling
ASTROPHYSICS James Binney
ATHEISM Julian Baggini
THE ATMOSPHERE Paul I. Palmer
AUGUSTINE Henry Chadwick
AUSTRALIA Kenneth Morgan
AUTISM Uta Frith
THE AVANT GARDE David Cottington
THE AZTECS Davíd Carrasco
BABYLONIA Trevor Bryce
BACTERIA Sebastian G. B. Amyes
BANKING John Goddard and
    John O. S. Wilson
BARTHES Jonathan Culler
THE BEATS David Sterritt
BEAUTY Roger Scruton
BEHAVIOURAL ECONOMICS
    Michelle Baddeley
BESTSELLERS John Sutherland
THE BIBLE John Riches
BIBLICAL ARCHAEOLOGY
    Eric H. Cline
BIOGRAPHY Hermione Lee
BLACK HOLES Katherine Blundell
BLOOD Chris Cooper
THE BLUES Elijah Wald
THE BODY Chris Shilling
THE BOOK OF MORMON
    Terryl Givens
BORDERS Alexander C. Diener
    and Joshua Hagen
THE BRAIN Michael O'Shea
BRANDING Robert Jones
THE BRICS Andrew F. Cooper
THE BRITISH CONSTITUTION
    Martin Loughlin
THE BRITISH EMPIRE Ashley Jackson
BRITISH POLITICS Anthony Wright
BUDDHA Michael Carrithers
BUDDHISM Damien Keown
BUDDHIST ETHICS Damien Keown
BYZANTIUM Peter Sarris
CALVINISM Jon Balserak
CANCER Nicholas James
CAPITALISM James Fulcher
CATHOLICISM Gerald O'Collins
CAUSATION Stephen Mumford and
    Rani Lill Anjum

THE CELL Terence Allen and
    Graham Cowling
THE CELTS Barry Cunliffe
CHAOS Leonard Smith
CHEMISTRY Peter Atkins
CHILD PSYCHOLOGY Usha Goswami
CHILDREN'S LITERATURE
    Kimberley Reynolds
CHINESE LITERATURE Sabina Knight
CHOICE THEORY Michael Allingham
CHRISTIAN ART Beth Williamson
CHRISTIAN ETHICS D. Stephen Long
CHRISTIANITY Linda Woodhead
CIRCADIAN RHYTHMS
    Russell Foster and Leon Kreitzman
CITIZENSHIP Richard Bellamy
CIVIL ENGINEERING
    David Muir Wood
CLASSICAL LITERATURE William Allan
CLASSICAL MYTHOLOGY
    Helen Morales
CLASSICS Mary Beard and
    John Henderson
CLAUSEWITZ Michael Howard
CLIMATE Mark Maslin
CLIMATE CHANGE Mark Maslin
CLINICAL PSYCHOLOGY
    Susan Llewelyn and
    Katie Aafjes-van Doorn
COGNITIVE NEUROSCIENCE
    Richard Passingham
THE COLD WAR Robert McMahon
COLONIAL AMERICA Alan Taylor
COLONIAL LATIN AMERICAN
    LITERATURE Rolena Adorno
COMBINATORICS Robin Wilson
COMEDY Matthew Bevis
COMMUNISM Leslie Holmes
COMPLEXITY John H. Holland
THE COMPUTER Darrel Ince
COMPUTER SCIENCE
    Subrata Dasgupta
CONFUCIANISM Daniel K. Gardner
THE CONQUISTADORS
    Matthew Restall and
    Felipe Fernández-Armesto
CONSCIENCE Paul Strohm
CONSCIOUSNESS Susan Blackmore
CONTEMPORARY ART
    Julian Stallabrass

CONTEMPORARY FICTION
    Robert Eaglestone
CONTINENTAL PHILOSOPHY
    Simon Critchley
COPERNICUS Owen Gingerich
CORAL REEFS Charles Sheppard
CORPORATE SOCIAL
    RESPONSIBILITY Jeremy Moon
CORRUPTION Leslie Holmes
COSMOLOGY Peter Coles
CRIME FICTION Richard Bradford
CRIMINAL JUSTICE Julian V. Roberts
CRITICAL THEORY
    Stephen Eric Bronner
THE CRUSADES Christopher Tyerman
CRYPTOGRAPHY Fred Piper and
    Sean Murphy
CRYSTALLOGRAPHY A. M. Glazer
THE CULTURAL REVOLUTION
    Richard Curt Kraus
DADA AND SURREALISM
    David Hopkins
DANTE Peter Hainsworth and
    David Robey
DARWIN Jonathan Howard
THE DEAD SEA SCROLLS
    Timothy H. Lim
DECOLONIZATION Dane Kennedy
DEMOCRACY Bernard Crick
DEPRESSION
    Jan Scott and Mary Jane Tacchi
DERRIDA Simon Glendinning
DESCARTES Tom Sorell
DESERTS Nick Middleton
DESIGN John Heskett
DEVELOPMENTAL BIOLOGY
    Lewis Wolpert
THE DEVIL Darren Oldridge
DIASPORA Kevin Kenny
DICTIONARIES Lynda Mugglestone
DINOSAURS David Norman
DIPLOMACY Joseph M. Siracusa
DOCUMENTARY FILM
    Patricia Aufderheide
DREAMING J. Allan Hobson
DRUGS Les Iversen
DRUIDS Barry Cunliffe
EARLY MUSIC Thomas Forrest Kelly
THE EARTH Martin Redfern
EARTH SYSTEM SCIENCE Tim Lenton

ECONOMICS Partha Dasgupta
EDUCATION Gary Thomas
EGYPTIAN MYTH Geraldine Pinch
EIGHTEENTH-CENTURY BRITAIN
    Paul Langford
THE ELEMENTS Philip Ball
EMOTION Dylan Evans
EMPIRE Stephen Howe
ENGELS Terrell Carver
ENGINEERING David Blockley
ENGLISH LITERATURE Jonathan Bate
THE ENLIGHTENMENT
    John Robertson
ENTREPRENEURSHIP Paul Westhead
    and Mike Wright
ENVIRONMENTAL ECONOMICS
    Stephen Smith
ENVIRONMENTAL POLITICS
    Andrew Dobson
EPICUREANISM Catherine Wilson
EPIDEMIOLOGY Rodolfo Saracci
ETHICS Simon Blackburn
ETHNOMUSICOLOGY Timothy Rice
THE ETRUSCANS Christopher Smith
EUGENICS Philippa Levine
THE EUROPEAN UNION
    John Pinder and Simon Usherwood
EUROPEAN UNION LAW
    Anthony Arnull
EVOLUTION
    Brian and Deborah Charlesworth
EXISTENTIALISM Thomas Flynn
EXPLORATION Stewart A. Weaver
THE EYE Michael Land
FAMILY LAW Jonathan Herring
FASCISM Kevin Passmore
FASHION Rebecca Arnold
FEMINISM Margaret Walters
FILM Michael Wood
FILM MUSIC Kathryn Kalinak
THE FIRST WORLD WAR
    Michael Howard
FOLK MUSIC Mark Slobin
FOOD John Krebs
FORENSIC PSYCHOLOGY
    David Canter
FORENSIC SCIENCE Jim Fraser
FORESTS Jaboury Ghazoul
FOSSILS Keith Thomson
FOUCAULT Gary Gutting

THE FOUNDING FATHERS
R. B. Bernstein
FRACTALS Kenneth Falconer
FREE SPEECH Nigel Warburton
FREE WILL Thomas Pink
FRENCH LITERATURE John D. Lyons
THE FRENCH REVOLUTION
William Doyle
FREUD Anthony Storr
FUNDAMENTALISM Malise Ruthven
FUNGI Nicholas P. Money
THE FUTURE Jennifer M. Gidley
GALAXIES John Gribbin
GALILEO Stillman Drake
GAME THEORY Ken Binmore
GANDHI Bhikhu Parekh
GENES Jonathan Slack
GENIUS Andrew Robinson
GEOGRAPHY John Matthews and
David Herbert
GEOPOLITICS Klaus Dodds
GERMAN LITERATURE Nicholas Boyle
GERMAN PHILOSOPHY
Andrew Bowie
GLOBAL CATASTROPHES Bill McGuire
GLOBAL ECONOMIC HISTORY
Robert C. Allen
GLOBALIZATION Manfred Steger
GOD John Bowker
GOETHE Ritchie Robertson
THE GOTHIC Nick Groom
GOVERNANCE Mark Bevir
GRAVITY Timothy Clifton
THE GREAT DEPRESSION AND
THE NEW DEAL Eric Rauchway
HABERMAS James Gordon Finlayson
THE HABSBURG EMPIRE
Martyn Rady
HAPPINESS Daniel M. Haybron
THE HARLEM RENAISSANCE
Cheryl A. Wall
THE HEBREW BIBLE AS LITERATURE
Tod Linafelt
HEGEL Peter Singer
HEIDEGGER Michael Inwood
HERMENEUTICS Jens Zimmermann
HERODOTUS Jennifer T. Roberts
HIEROGLYPHS Penelope Wilson
HINDUISM Kim Knott
HISTORY John H. Arnold

THE HISTORY OF ASTRONOMY
Michael Hoskin
THE HISTORY OF CHEMISTRY
William H. Brock
THE HISTORY OF LIFE
Michael Benton
THE HISTORY OF MATHEMATICS
Jacqueline Stedall
THE HISTORY OF MEDICINE
William Bynum
THE HISTORY OF TIME
Leofranc Holford-Strevens
HIV AND AIDS Alan Whiteside
HOBBES Richard Tuck
HOLLYWOOD Peter Decherney
HOME Michael Allen Fox
HORMONES Martin Luck
HUMAN ANATOMY
Leslie Klenerman
HUMAN EVOLUTION Bernard Wood
HUMAN RIGHTS Andrew Clapham
HUMANISM Stephen Law
HUME A. J. Ayer
HUMOUR Noël Carroll
THE ICE AGE Jamie Woodward
IDEOLOGY Michael Freeden
INDIAN CINEMA
Ashish Rajadhyaksha
INDIAN PHILOSOPHY Sue Hamilton
THE INDUSTRIAL REVOLUTION
Robert C. Allen
INFECTIOUS DISEASE Marta L. Wayne
and Benjamin M. Bolker
INFINITY Ian Stewart
INFORMATION Luciano Floridi
INNOVATION Mark Dodgson
and David Gann
INTELLIGENCE Ian J. Deary
INTELLECTUAL PROPERTY
Siva Vaidhyanathan
INTERNATIONAL LAW
Vaughan Lowe
INTERNATIONAL MIGRATION
Khalid Koser
INTERNATIONAL RELATIONS
Paul Wilkinson
INTERNATIONAL SECURITY
Christopher S. Browning
IRAN Ali M. Ansari
ISLAM Malise Ruthven

ISLAMIC HISTORY Adam Silverstein
ISOTOPES Rob Ellam
ITALIAN LITERATURE
    Peter Hainsworth and David Robey
JESUS Richard Bauckham
JEWISH HISTORY David N. Myers
JOURNALISM Ian Hargreaves
JUDAISM Norman Solomon
JUNG Anthony Stevens
KABBALAH Joseph Dan
KAFKA Ritchie Robertson
KANT Roger Scruton
KEYNES Robert Skidelsky
KIERKEGAARD Patrick Gardiner
KNOWLEDGE Jennifer Nagel
THE KORAN Michael Cook
LANDSCAPE ARCHITECTURE
    Ian H. Thompson
LANDSCAPES AND
    GEOMORPHOLOGY
    Andrew Goudie and Heather Viles
LANGUAGES Stephen R. Anderson
LATE ANTIQUITY Gillian Clark
LAW Raymond Wacks
THE LAWS OF THERMODYNAMICS
    Peter Atkins
LEADERSHIP Keith Grint
LEARNING Mark Haselgrove
LEIBNIZ Maria Rosa Antognazza
LIBERALISM Michael Freeden
LIGHT Ian Walmsley
LINCOLN Allen C. Guelzo
LINGUISTICS Peter Matthews
LITERARY THEORY Jonathan Culler
LOCKE John Dunn
LOGIC Graham Priest
LOVE Ronald de Sousa
MACHIAVELLI Quentin Skinner
MADNESS Andrew Scull
MAGIC Owen Davies
MAGNA CARTA Nicholas Vincent
MAGNETISM Stephen Blundell
MALTHUS Donald Winch
MANAGEMENT John Hendry
MAO Delia Davin
MARINE BIOLOGY Philip V. Mladenov
THE MARQUIS DE SADE John Phillips
MARTIN LUTHER Scott H. Hendrix
MARTYRDOM Jolyon Mitchell
MARX Peter Singer

MATERIALS Christopher Hall
MATHEMATICS Timothy Gowers
THE MEANING OF LIFE
    Terry Eagleton
MEASUREMENT David Hand
MEDICAL ETHICS Tony Hope
MEDICAL LAW Charles Foster
MEDIEVAL BRITAIN John Gillingham
    and Ralph A. Griffiths
MEDIEVAL LITERATURE
    Elaine Treharne
MEDIEVAL PHILOSOPHY
    John Marenbon
MEMORY Jonathan K. Foster
METAPHYSICS Stephen Mumford
THE MEXICAN REVOLUTION
    Alan Knight
MICHAEL FARADAY
    Frank A. J. L. James
MICROBIOLOGY Nicholas P. Money
MICROECONOMICS Avinash Dixit
MICROSCOPY Terence Allen
THE MIDDLE AGES Miri Rubin
MILITARY JUSTICE Eugene R. Fidell
MILITARY STRATEGY
    Antulio J. Echevarria II
MINERALS David Vaughan
MODERN ART David Cottington
MODERN CHINA Rana Mitter
MODERN DRAMA
    Kirsten E. Shepherd-Barr
MODERN FRANCE
    Vanessa R. Schwartz
MODERN IRELAND Senia Pašeta
MODERN ITALY Anna Cento Bull
MODERN JAPAN
    Christopher Goto-Jones
MODERN LATIN AMERICAN
    LITERATURE
    Roberto González Echevarría
MODERN WAR Richard English
MODERNISM Christopher Butler
MOLECULAR BIOLOGY
    Aysha Divan and Janice A. Royds
MOLECULES Philip Ball
THE MONGOLS Morris Rossabi
MOONS David A. Rothery
MORMONISM
    Richard Lyman Bushman
MOUNTAINS Martin F. Price

MUHAMMAD Jonathan A. C. Brown
MULTICULTURALISM Ali Rattansi
MULTILINGUALISM John C. Maher
MUSIC Nicholas Cook
MYTH Robert A. Segal
THE NAPOLEONIC WARS
    Mike Rapport
NATIONALISM Steven Grosby
NAVIGATION Jim Bennett
NELSON MANDELA Elleke Boehmer
NEOLIBERALISM Manfred Steger
    and Ravi Roy
NETWORKS Guido Caldarelli
    and Michele Catanzaro
THE NEW TESTAMENT
    Luke Timothy Johnson
THE NEW TESTAMENT AS
    LITERATURE Kyle Keefer
NEWTON Robert Iliffe
NIETZSCHE Michael Tanner
NINETEENTH-CENTURY BRITAIN
    Christopher Harvie and
    H. C. G. Matthew
THE NORMAN CONQUEST
    George Garnett
NORTH AMERICAN INDIANS
    Theda Perdue and Michael D. Green
NORTHERN IRELAND
    Marc Mulholland
NOTHING Frank Close
NUCLEAR PHYSICS Frank Close
NUCLEAR POWER Maxwell Irvine
NUCLEAR WEAPONS
    Joseph M. Siracusa
NUMBERS Peter M. Higgins
NUTRITION David A. Bender
OBJECTIVITY Stephen Gaukroger
THE OLD TESTAMENT
    Michael D. Coogan
THE ORCHESTRA D. Kern Holoman
ORGANIC CHEMISTRY
    Graham Patrick
ORGANIZATIONS Mary Jo Hatch
PAGANISM Owen Davies
PAIN Rob Boddice
THE PALESTINIAN-ISRAELI
    CONFLICT Martin Bunton
PANDEMICS Christian W. McMillen
PARTICLE PHYSICS Frank Close
PAUL E. P. Sanders

PEACE Oliver P. Richmond
PENTECOSTALISM William K. Kay
THE PERIODIC TABLE Eric R. Scerri
PHILOSOPHY Edward Craig
PHILOSOPHY IN THE ISLAMIC
    WORLD Peter Adamson
PHILOSOPHY OF LAW
    Raymond Wacks
PHILOSOPHY OF SCIENCE
    Samir Okasha
PHOTOGRAPHY Steve Edwards
PHYSICAL CHEMISTRY Peter Atkins
PILGRIMAGE Ian Reader
PLAGUE Paul Slack
PLANETS David A. Rothery
PLANTS Timothy Walker
PLATE TECTONICS Peter Molnar
PLATO Julia Annas
POLITICAL PHILOSOPHY
    David Miller
POLITICS Kenneth Minogue
POPULISM Cas Mudde and
    Cristóbal Rovira Kaltwasser
POSTCOLONIALISM Robert Young
POSTMODERNISM Christopher Butler
POSTSTRUCTURALISM
    Catherine Belsey
PREHISTORY Chris Gosden
PRESOCRATIC PHILOSOPHY
    Catherine Osborne
PRIVACY Raymond Wacks
PROBABILITY John Haigh
PROGRESSIVISM Walter Nugent
PROTESTANTISM Mark A. Noll
PSYCHIATRY Tom Burns
PSYCHOANALYSIS Daniel Pick
PSYCHOLOGY
    Gillian Butler and Freda McManus
PSYCHOTHERAPY Tom Burns and
    Eva Burns-Lundgren
PUBLIC ADMINISTRATION
    Stella Z. Theodoulou and Ravi K. Roy
PUBLIC HEALTH Virginia Berridge
PURITANISM Francis J. Bremer
THE QUAKERS Pink Dandelion
QUANTUM THEORY
    John Polkinghorne
RACISM Ali Rattansi
RADIOACTIVITY Claudio Tuniz
RASTAFARI Ennis B. Edmonds

THE REAGAN REVOLUTION Gil Troy
REALITY Jan Westerhoff
THE REFORMATION Peter Marshall
RELATIVITY Russell Stannard
RELIGION IN AMERICA Timothy Beal
THE RENAISSANCE Jerry Brotton
RENAISSANCE ART
   Geraldine A. Johnson
REVOLUTIONS Jack A. Goldstone
RHETORIC Richard Toye
RISK Baruch Fischhoff and John Kadvany
RITUAL Barry Stephenson
RIVERS Nick Middleton
ROBOTICS Alan Winfield
ROCKS Jan Zalasiewicz
ROMAN BRITAIN Peter Salway
THE ROMAN EMPIRE
   Christopher Kelly
THE ROMAN REPUBLIC
   David M. Gwynn
ROMANTICISM Michael Ferber
ROUSSEAU Robert Wokler
RUSSELL A. C. Grayling
RUSSIAN HISTORY Geoffrey Hosking
RUSSIAN LITERATURE Catriona Kelly
THE RUSSIAN REVOLUTION
   S. A. Smith
SAVANNAS Peter A. Furley
SCHIZOPHRENIA Chris Frith and
   Eve Johnstone
SCHOPENHAUER
   Christopher Janaway
SCIENCE AND RELIGION
   Thomas Dixon
SCIENCE FICTION David Seed
THE SCIENTIFIC REVOLUTION
   Lawrence M. Principe
SCOTLAND Rab Houston
SEXUALITY Véronique Mottier
SHAKESPEARE'S COMEDIES
   Bart van Es
SHAKESPEARE'S TRAGEDIES
   Stanley Wells
SIKHISM Eleanor Nesbitt
THE SILK ROAD James A. Millward
SLANG Jonathon Green
SLEEP Steven W. Lockley and
   Russell G. Foster
SOCIAL AND CULTURAL
   ANTHROPOLOGY
   John Monaghan and Peter Just

SOCIAL PSYCHOLOGY Richard J. Crisp
SOCIAL WORK Sally Holland and
   Jonathan Scourfield
SOCIALISM Michael Newman
SOCIOLINGUISTICS John Edwards
SOCIOLOGY Steve Bruce
SOCRATES C. C. W. Taylor
SOUND Mike Goldsmith
THE SOVIET UNION Stephen Lovell
THE SPANISH CIVIL WAR
   Helen Graham
SPANISH LITERATURE Jo Labanyi
SPINOZA Roger Scruton
SPIRITUALITY Philip Sheldrake
SPORT Mike Cronin
STARS Andrew King
STATISTICS David J. Hand
STEM CELLS Jonathan Slack
STRUCTURAL ENGINEERING
   David Blockley
STUART BRITAIN John Morrill
SUPERCONDUCTIVITY
   Stephen Blundell
SYMMETRY Ian Stewart
TAXATION Stephen Smith
TEETH Peter S. Ungar
TELESCOPES Geoff Cottrell
TERRORISM Charles Townshend
THEATRE Marvin Carlson
THEOLOGY David F. Ford
THOMAS AQUINAS Fergus Kerr
THOUGHT Tim Bayne
TIBETAN BUDDHISM
   Matthew T. Kapstein
TOCQUEVILLE Harvey C. Mansfield
TRAGEDY Adrian Poole
TRANSLATION Matthew Reynolds
THE TROJAN WAR Eric H. Cline
TRUST Katherine Hawley
THE TUDORS John Guy
TWENTIETH-CENTURY BRITAIN
   Kenneth O. Morgan
THE UNITED NATIONS
   Jussi M. Hanhimäki
THE U.S. CONGRESS Donald A. Ritchie
THE U.S. SUPREME COURT
   Linda Greenhouse
UTOPIANISM Lyman Tower Sargent
THE VIKINGS Julian Richards
VIRUSES Dorothy H. Crawford
VOLTAIRE Nicholas Cronk

WAR AND TECHNOLOGY
    Alex Roland
WATER John Finney
WEATHER Storm Dunlop
THE WELFARE STATE
    David Garland
WILLIAM SHAKESPEARE
    Stanley Wells
WITCHCRAFT Malcolm Gaskill

WITTGENSTEIN A. C. Grayling
WORK Stephen Fineman
WORLD MUSIC Philip Bohlman
THE WORLD TRADE
    ORGANIZATION Amrita Narlikar
WORLD WAR II Gerhard L. Weinberg
WRITING AND SCRIPT
    Andrew Robinson
ZIONISM Michael Stanislawski

Available soon:

OCEANS Dorrik Stow
UTILITARIANISM
    Katarzyna de Lazari-Radek and
    Peter Singer

THE UNIVERSITY
    David Palfreyman and Paul Temple
HEREDITY John Waller
FREEMASONRY Andreas Önnerfors

For more information visit our website

www.oup.com/vsi/

Rob Boddice

PAIN

A Very Short Introduction

OXFORD
UNIVERSITY PRESS

OXFORD
UNIVERSITY PRESS

Great Clarendon Street, Oxford, OX2 6DP,
United Kingdom

Oxford University Press is a department of the University of Oxford.
It furthers the University's objective of excellence in research, scholarship,
and education by publishing worldwide. Oxford is a registered trade mark of
Oxford University Press in the UK and in certain other countries

Published in the United States of America by Oxford University Press
198 Madison Avenue, New York, NY 10016, United States of America

British Library Cataloguing in Publication Data
Data available

Library of Congress Control Number: 2017930570

ISBN 978-0-19-873856-5

Printed in Great Britain by
Ashford Colour Press Ltd, Gosport, Hampshire

Contents

Acknowledgements xv

List of illustrations xvii

Introduction 1

1 Pain concepts 5

2 Pain and piety 15

3 Pain and the machine 27

4 Pain and civilization 43

5 Sympathy, compassion, empathy 53

6 Pain as pleasure 65

7 Pain in modern medicine and science 77

8 Chronic pain 94

9 Cultures of pain 105

References 119

Further reading 123

Index 127

Acknowledgements

I've been in a world of pain for several years, and could not have come through it without significant personal, professional, and institutional support. The immediate impetus for writing this book came from Mary Cosgrove, who was visiting the Center for the History of Emotions at the Max Planck Institute for Human Development in Berlin. Most of the book has been written under the roof of that Institute, with generous support in particular from Ute Frevert. Much of the research took place in the Osler Library for the History of Medicine at McGill University in Montreal. I would not have been well placed to write such a book without the invitation to take up a fellowship at the Birkbeck Pain Project in 2012, under the guidance of Joanna Bourke. The conference I organized for the Pain Project has helped guide my holistic and multi-disciplinary view of pain, as well as introducing me to a host of pain scholars from across the intellectual map. I am in the debt of the contributors to my edited volume, *Pain and Emotion in Modern History*. Along the way, I also received invaluable insights from Daniel Goldberg, Imke Rajamani, Frederik Schröer, and Michael Weinman, as well as the members of the Melbourne node of the Australian Research Council Centre of Excellence for the History of Emotions. Tony Morris helped make this book happen. Latha Menon at Oxford University Press encouraged the project, and was instrumental in improving the manuscript. Thanks to the Deutsche Forschungsgemeinschaft for funding my pain research, and to Martin Lücke for hosting me with such professional cordiality at Freie Universität Berlin. In addition to being emotional, moral, and intellectual support throughout the writing process, Stephanie Olsen has also unintentionally afforded me first-hand experience of living with someone with chronic pain. It is my profound hope that the publication of this volume signals a release of pain, in every sense.

Pain

List of illustrations

1   Bernard Picart, *The Death of Hercules* (1731) **8**
    Rijksmuseum, Amsterdam

2   Geertgen tot Sint Jans, *Christus als Man van smarten* (*c.*1486) **16**
    Museum Catharijneconvent, Utrecht, photo Ruben de Heer

3   Christ on the Cross (17th century), Holy Roman Empire, from the Deutsches Historisches Museum **19**
    Deutsches Historisches Museum, Berlin / A. Psille

4   Gerard David, *Judgement of Cambyses* (1488) **22**
    Heritage Image Partnership Ltd / Alamy Stock Photo

5   The Pain Pathway, from René Descartes, *Traite de l'homme* (1664) **29**
    Wellcome Library, London

6   Algometer, from Cesare Lombroso, *Criminal Man* (1911) **36**
    Wellcome Library, London

7   Hysterical woman yawning, Nouvelle iconographie de la Salpêtrière (1890) **51**
    Wellcome Library, London

8   Richard von Kraft-Ebing, *Man on all fours in red jacket with clothed woman riding him and holding a whip* (*c.*1896) **71**
    Wellcome Library, London

9   Gate control mechanism (1965) **81**
    From Melzack, Wall, 'Pain Mechanisms: A New Theory', Science 1965, figure 4. Reprinted with permission from AAAS. http://science.sciencemag.org/content/150/3699/971

10 Social and physical pain produce similar brain responses **89**
    Reprinted from *NeuroImage*, 22/1, Matthew D. Lieberman, Johanna M. Jarcho, Steve Berman, Bruce D. Naliboff, Brandall Y. Suyenobu, Mark Mandelkern, Emeran A. Mayer, The neural correlates of placebo effects: a disruption account, Pages No. 447–55, Copyright (2004), with permission from Elsevier

11 Charles Bell, *Opisthotonos* (1809) **109**

© The Royal College of Surgeons of Edinburgh

12 Rudolf Saudek, *Death Mask of Nietzsche* (*c.*1910) **115**

© Saudek, Rudolf (b.1880) / Private Collection / Archives Charmet / Bridgeman Images

13 Francis Bacon, *Three Studies for a Crucifixion* (1962) **116**

Three Studies for a Crucifixion, March 1962, by Francis Bacon. The Solomon R. Guggenheim Foundation / Art. Resource, NY / Scala, Florence. © DACS 2017

Pain

Introduction

What is pain? It is all too easy to assume that everybody already knows the answer to this question. We've all stubbed a toe, put a thumb between hammer and nail, or had a headache. Countless millions know what it is to have back pain. Millions of others know about cancer pain and the pain caused by treating it. Intuitively, pain would seem to be implicitly understood but resistant to attempts at description. It may suffice for many to simply acknowledge that pain *is*, and leave it at that.

For many others, however, and not least for the medical community, pain remains enigmatic, mysterious, and frustrating. The International Association for the Study of Pain (IASP) is a non-profit society founded in 1973 by John Bonica (1917–94). Bonica pioneered research into pain management in the United States after an early career as a professional wrestler that caused his own lifelong chronic pain conditions. The IASP was to promote pain research in the field of medicine, broadly defined. Its current 'official' definition of pain, and the guiding principle for publications in its journal, *Pain*, is as follows: 'Pain is an unpleasant sensory and emotional experience associated with actual or potential tissue damage or described in terms of such damage'. For a whole variety of reasons, this definition is thought by many to be inadequate, and even misleading. Pain is unpredictable and resistant to standards of measurement and treatment. It gets bundled up with confusing social and cultural factors. For those with injuries of various severities, it often appears when it technically shouldn't, and fails to appear when one would have assumed it would. Then there are those who suffer with chronic pain, whose complaints have been difficult to correlate with any particular injury or lesion, or even allusions to such, and for whom medication seems to be of no help. Moreover, people complain of pain even where there is no injury. Feelings *hurt*. Hearts *break*. Do such phrases hint at a deeper understanding of how pain works and what pain means? A multidisciplinary account of pain shows that attempts to fix a definition belie the fluid nature of pain itself.

Pain has become one of the most challenging medical mysteries of modern times, in terms of how it works (pain mechanisms), how to treat it (pain management), and what it means (pain experience). Enormous strides have been taken in recent decades concerning our understanding of both physical and emotional pain. Contemporary pain specialists aver a 'biopsychosocial' model of pain, in which the body and mind are bound up with social factors that add up to our collective pain experiences. No account of pain that eliminates any one or more of these three factors—biological, psychological, social—will afford a satisfactory understanding of painful phenomena. Yet for most of the modern medical history of pain, the psychological element was abstracted as an irrational modifier of physical signs. All too commonly, chronic pain sufferers had their 'character' called into question because doctors could not find sufficient physical causes of their distress. And if psychological factors were underplayed or misunderstood, social and cultural factors were, until quite recently, more or less ignored. What makes this surprising is that, throughout history, and all across the world, most sufferers of pain shared a biopsychosocial understanding of their plight, even if they could not quite articulate it as such.

Because of this, my *Very Short Introduction* to pain takes a very long view. There is a massive store of knowledge about pain, much of it historical, which helps situate contemporary medical accounts. To understand pain as it is, one must understand the vast possibilities of pain experience. It cannot be reduced axiomatically because it is always contextually situated. How we communicate—that is, the labels we give to pain—and how we conceptualize—that is, the ways in which we *see* pain, especially in others—are essential to the ways in which pain is experienced. This book will come to a discussion of bodies, nerves, neuroscience, and functional magnetic resonance imaging (fMRI). It will come to a discussion of endogenous opioids and the reasons why an over-the-counter pain pill works. But none of this will make sense without first introducing the languages, cultures, and historical variabilities of pain. And once introduced, they do not disappear as mechanistic views arise, but remain sometimes to challenge and sometimes to complement such views.

Nor does this book dwell entirely on first-hand pain. Both the history of pain and current medical investigations of pain have had to tackle the question of how we conceive, understand, and experience the pain of others. What is it to see pain? What does sympathy or empathy with pain depend on? Is empathic pain, in fact, really the same as first-hand pain? These questions are part and parcel of contemporary approaches to pain that seek continually to entangle the physical and the emotional, the body and the mind, and the brain and the world.

This holistic focus keeps us grounded in worlds of pain, where expression is as important as, and sometimes a complicating factor to, both experience and a science of sensitivity. It is necessary to look at pain, not only to see what it is in a positive, physiological sense, but also in order to reflect on what we commonly know about it. To see pain, suffering, anguish, grief is, most of the time, to understand it and to enter into it.

But sometimes it is obscure, alien, or incomprehensible to us. Conversely, sometimes we see what we think is pain, but find on closer examination that there is none at all.

Pain is conveyed in a multitude of ways, from screams to silence, and from gritted teeth to tears. Pain famously employs metaphors, of weapons and the terrible wounds they do, but people are too imaginative to rely on words and utterances alone. Pain has been painted, sculpted, captured on film. It has reached out from the walls of galleries and collapsed the distance between the artist's pain and the viewer's implicit knowledge about what that must feel like. If humans are empathic creatures—if people truly have the capacity for empathy—then it must be acknowledged that in particular, contextually defined, and culturally specific ways, we are constantly surrounded by expressions of pain. That we understand this world of pain so implicitly is part of the mystery of pain that humans, as a species, have sought to explain. We continue on that path.

Pain

Chapter 1
Pain concepts

Scour the shelves of a specialist library on the history of medicine, looking for pain. It will strike you, as it struck me in the Osler Library in Montreal, that there are many more books on the history of anaesthesia than there are on the history of pain. Triumphs and conquests of pain abound in the modern celebration of medical science's ability to benumb. Yet there's something uncanny about this celebration, for the starting point for many of these works on anaesthesia is the claim that, until the mid-19th century, pain was central to the experience of being human. Pain, along with death, was a certainty in life. The history of pain, therefore, dwarfs the history of anaesthesia. Even now, in the age of the pain killer, all our efforts to make pain go away are haunted by the persistence and tenacity of pain. For when pain killers wear off, pain remains, either in fact or in potentia. To the extent that we still produce an endless stream of books and articles about anaesthesia, and about pain management, we implicitly acknowledge that pain still is a certainty.

Vocabularies of pain

The first thing to say about pain is that we are not dealing with a timeless, simply mechanical phenomenon. Pain has been many things, in many places. While this Introduction to pain will culminate with contemporary Western medicine's current understandings of, and practices concerning, pain, to get there first requires an account of pain that might seem unfamiliar or strange. We must understand the vocabulary of pain and the historical conceptual range of pain. The single word 'pain', in English, does not suffice. Modern English has separated out pain (a physical feeling of hurt) from suffering, with all of the latter's emotional connotations. We might commonly re-introduce a conceptual slippage by talking about hurt feelings or the pain of grief, but modern medical discourse has striven for carefully marked conceptual labels. This is, perhaps, in the process of changing. But let us turn to antiquity and imagine a world in which there is no clear distinction between pains of the body and pains of what we might call an emotional nature. These pains of the soul, generalized sufferings, or passions, could be as painful as a war wound, and perhaps even more so.

The ancient Greeks had a number of words for pain and suffering that tended to overlap. Chief among these terms was *algos*, which denoted physical pain as well as woe, ill, or misery. The wrath of Achilles, according to Homer, brought these upon the Achaeans, and indeed it is impossible in the Homeric epic to disentangle suffering from pain, unless it is to contrast the lasting significance of suffering at the level of the soul from the passing anguish of the body. Modern concepts that favour a dualistic tradition of mind and body do no more justice to the Greek *algos* as our separation of the concepts of speech and thought does to *logos*. The dualistic tradition, its influence and its shortcomings, will frequently detain us, and is central to an understanding of pain in Western modernity. Yet it is perhaps better to think in the vernacular, rather than in the specialized terminology of medicine or philosophy. In English, when we are slighted, or crushed in defeat, or disappointed in love, we talk of 'hurt' and 'pain', just as Homer would have done. Twentieth-century specialists in the treatment of pain in particular tended to dismiss such talk as metaphor, but there is a literal truth to a linguistic trait that has been sustained since antiquity. If I fall and break my arm while out walking in the forest, I might complain that it hurts, but whatever the nature of my physical pain, that hurt will always also express fear, alarm, and an agitated state of planning for action. Similarly, a husband who hears of the loss of his family in a car accident will say he is in pain. He should be believed.

The Greeks did have a way of isolating bodily pain, if necessary, although it was only ever a short elision to a more general concept of suffering. In the *Iliad*, talk of *odune* is never far away from the general state of anguish that undergirds the epic, and the same is true of the famous Herculean scream in Sophocles' (d. 406 BCE) *Trachiniae*. The poisoned robe that slowly kills the hero in a prolonged fit of agony puts Heracles interchangeably in bodily pain and woeful misery (*odune* and *algos*). Mythic accounts have him throw himself on his self-built funeral pyre and burn to 'heal' his suffering (see Figure 1). If the categories aren't confusing enough, the generic Greek term from which we derive 'passion' also denotes suffering, although some careful caveats have to be introduced here. The Greek term *pathos* denotes suffering or experience and, in its original meaning, the adjective 'pathetic' was an appeal at an emotional level. In Aristotle's (384–322 BCE) rhetoric, pathos causes pleasure or pain in an audience, as well as in its producer, depending on which emotions are mobilized. The possibility of pain without injury is clear, and it is closely entangled with affective states. Aristotle goes so far as to say that the person who is angry 'suffers pain'. Here we see the elision of grief or vexation with bodily pain in the word *lupé*.

The Latin derivation of pathos, through *pashein*, is the word *passio*. The conflation of the emotional and the physical, of suffering and pain, is continued. It is easy to forget the physical element here, since the English word 'passion' seems predominantly to refer to a form of emotional enthusiasm, such as might be found in the 'passionate' supporter of a football team. Actually, this oversight is strange. Head into any church and you'll find the stations of the cross, depicting Christ's passion. The word here clearly denotes

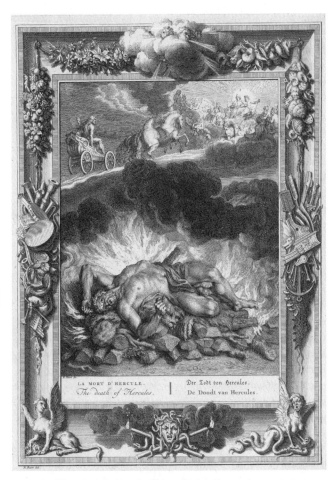

1. **Bernard Picart,** *The Death of Hercules* (1731).

Christ's *suffering*. There will be more to say about this, but for now it suffices to say that the Roman world preserved a Greek comingling of emotional and physical suffering. Nowhere was this clearer than among the Stoics, whose philosophy was widespread from the 3rd century BCE, beginning in Athens, until Justinian

8

(483–565 CE) put an end to pagan philosophy in 529 CE. Since behaviour was the chief indicator of virtue for the Stoics, so-called 'irrational' (*alogos*) passions were to be shut down or closed off. According to Diogenes Laertius (3rd century CE), the irrational passions that caused movements of the soul contrary to nature included fear and grief, and therefore pain. All were considered irrational contractions (of the mind). The Stoic life was a life that not only suppressed or controlled emotion, but also refused to acknowledge, or pay attention to, pain. Indeed, the two were scarcely distinguishable. Consider Diogenes Laertius' phrase from his *Lives of Eminent Philosophers*: 'pity is grief [bodily pain] felt at undeserved suffering [distress]', and the holistic experience of bodily pain and passion emerges, not so much in clarity as in a complex mixture of types of experience at the level of the soul.

If the Romans emphasized the emotional level of pain through *passio*, they also, like the Greeks, had a generally holistic approach to the concept of pain that included what has more recently been divided into mental and physical categories. The Latin *dolor* is preserved in the French *douleur*, the Spanish *dolor*, and the Italian *dolore*. It could stand for physical pain, as well as grief, anguish, sorrow, and resentment. To some extent, the conflation has been preserved, but most European languages make a clear distinction between physical and mental pain (*souffrance*, *sufrimiento*, and *sofferenza*, respectively in the three languages just mentioned). This is also true in German, where the etymologically distinct words *Schmerz* and *Leid* clearly distinguish the body from the mind.

Conceptual ambiguities

If anything, contemporary European categories of pain suffer from the compound confusions of their etymologies. Galen of Pergamon (129–200/216 CE) was an enormously influential physician and surgeon who bequeathed to us the language of temperament (literally, 'mixture', from the Latin *tempere*). Humans were made up of four humours: blood or sanguis, phlegm, yellow bile or *kholé*, and black bile or *melaina kholé*. Each of the humours was related to a natural element, air, water, fire and earth, respectively, and an imbalance of humours in the body had a profound effect on the nature of the individual. Humoral imbalance was a sign of illness and a cause of pain. Galenism, departing from the Stoics and Aristotelian philosophy, conflates the spiritual and the bodily, collapsing distinctions of material and immaterial.

Humorism was profoundly influential in the history of medicine, and inspired physiological thinking until the 19th century. Even now, the linguistic legacy remains with us. The disease of cholera takes its name from an excess of yellow bile, transliterated from Greek into Latin. Yet in French and Spanish, *colère* and *cólera* mean 'anger'. According to Aristotle, and later Seneca, anger was conceived as a feeling of pain, intermixed with a desire for revenge. Thanks to Galenism, however, what we might commonly think of as an immaterial emotion has been, for most of its history, conceived of as rooted in the body.

Similarly, an excess of black bile has given us 'melancholy', which proved to be a remarkably unstable category of pathological disorder. Robert Burton's (1577–1640) *Anatomy of Melancholy* (1621), for example, leaves no doubt about the bodily suffering caused by many types of melancholy, which were nevertheless experienced as a passionate malaise. In modernity, melancholy was a forerunner of depression (which is a distinctly recent diagnostic category), but if the pathology has shifted to the mind, it nevertheless retains its ability to physically incapacitate with pain. A phlegmatic temperament originally had an excess of phlegm and might be bilious, but is now considered to be stoical or apathetic. Galen mentioned that this humour had to be evacuated or else it caused great pain (a lot of grief). To be sanguine, however, in contemporary parlance, is to be an optimist despite indications of difficulty. Such people are often referred to as 'ruddy': a description of the excess of blood in their faces that somehow indicates their positivity.

Bodily pain in general could be ascribed to an imbalance of humours (ailments that could be closely associated with behaviour and practice, hence the virtue of temperance and the vice of intemperance). To take just two examples, Esther Cohen, in *The Modulated Scream* (2010), documented the description of types of pain by Maurus of Salerno in the late 12th century, which connected specific humours with specific orders of pain. Stretching pain (*extensivus*) related to black bile; stabbing pain (*pungitivus*) to yellow bile; a chaining or restraining pain (*aggravativus*) was related to phlegm; and a fixed or pressing pain (*infixivus*) was related to blood. And Jan Frans van Dijkhuizen, in *The Sense of Suffering* (2009), illuminated Gualterus Breule's 1632 work, *Praxis medicinae*, which understood headache as the result of 'swelling humours ascending from the lower Parts', resulting, fittingly enough, in 'painefull griefe'.

For a good chunk of late modernity, doctors thought the vagaries of the vernacular were reason enough to mistrust patient testimony about pain, preferring mechanical measuring innovations to try to establish the nature of afflictions objectively. The IASP official definition of pain that I alluded to in the Introduction was taken from Harold Merskey, who had himself traced some of the ancient languages and concepts of pain. Yet despite finding conceptual slippages among pain, sorrow, and grief, he concluded that these amounted to translation error, so that two ideas, pain and emotion, have been treated 'as if they were identical, an error which seems to have beset the notion of pain in nearly every century'. Several millennia of common knowledge were overridden in order to narrow the definition of pain (whether sensory or emotional) to something to do with injury. There are good reasons to assume that Galenic categories, though outmoded and debunked from the point of view of contemporary biology, do in fact communicate something about the body in pain that 20th-century biology in particular resisted. Just as with other ancient nomenclature concerning pain and suffering, modern languages retain a concept of the individual whose sufferings are not readily distinguishable as mental and physical, but are taken together holistically, and do not necessarily have anything to do with injury.

Thinking globally about pain

The categorical vernacular conflation is not limited to Western civilization (which in any case was never sealed off from encounters with so-called 'non-Western' influences). As Paolo Santangelo has shown for Late Imperial China, for example, there is a rich overlapping of physical, emotional, sensational, and moral categories, with an interplay of characters such as *tong*, *ku*, and the portmanteau *tongku*, denoting respectively 'painful', 'suffering', and, together, something like 'anguish'. In contemporary China, pain is related to a stagnation of *ch'i* (*qi*)—the cosmological energy field—manifested as congealed blood, which is implicated as much in sharp pain as in anxiety. The relationship is marked in linguistic tradition, with *t'ong* meaning pain and *tōng* meaning flow. It is to the restoration of flow that acupuncture is intended. The Chinese understanding of pain, stemming from Taoist and Confucian traditions, is holistic, meaning that pain is inherent in being human just as being human is cosmologically inseparable from all that is. Nevertheless, as Wei-Ming Tu has put it, humans 'experience pain more acutely and suffer more intensely' than anything else in existence because humans are 'the most sentient and therefore the most vulnerable emotionally, most responsive psychologically and most sensible intellectually'. The notion of a mind/body dualism or a separation of physical and emotional pain simply makes no sense in traditional Chinese thinking.

In India, the Hindi word *dard* stands for a raft of different degrees of suffering, from uneasiness to torture and from mental distress to grief to anguish. When the protagonist of the 1985 film *Mard* (Man/Macho) declares 'Jo mard hotā hai usse darḍ nahin hotā' (he who is a real man feels no pain), he does so with reference to the cutting or whipping of the body and to cut short the lacrimonious onset of grief for his dead mother. A correlate would be the word *duḥkh*, which often translates as sorrow or grief, but which can signify pain just the same. It has ancient roots in Sanskrit, connoting suffering on a spiritual level, but when deployed in compound terms can indicate the whole range of pain from a cut to a cramp to a calamity. The word was used frequently by the Bengali Nobel Laureate Rabrindranath Tagore (1861–1941), to give a sense of trouble or grief or pain in the everyday.

In Arabic, the generic word ألم (*'alam*) works as well for pain as for suffering, for ache as for misery. The correlation runs deeper. Linguistic scholar Zouhair Maalej has noted the conceptual, symbolic, and embodied interconnection of anger and physical pain in Tunisian Arabic, for example. In general, in the Islamic world, pain is seen as a predestined part of God's will, which, though it by no means precludes seeking its relief, reminds the sufferer of the Creator and the need for patience, endurance, and faith. Traditionally, the treatment of pain in the Islamic world is not opposed to medicinal or analgesic cures, but the focus is on the spiritual core of the individual, on prayer, on reading the Koran, and on the contemplation of the divine. All these things aid in changing the focus of attention away from suffering. In the mid-1980s, Islamic physician Mohamed Al-Jeilani noted that Western pain management's (reluctant) turn to the psyche—to emotions as the key to the understanding and relief of pain—had been taken by Islamic scholars centuries ago.

Taken together, this survey only begins to scratch the surface of languages and concepts of pain, a global and historical study of which could fill volumes. I begin with this semantic journey to emphasize both an enduring conceptual continuity in the understanding of pain and a seismic rupture in this understanding that radically altered what it meant to be in pain, to be treated for pain (or ignored), and to treat for pain (medically) in Western modernity, particularly after Descartes. That rupture also indicates a historic separation of vernacular knowledge of pain from medical specialism about pain. What should be clear immediately, however, is that pain resists—indeed, it has always resisted—a narrow definition. Even the etymology of the English word 'pain', deriving from the Latin *poena*, indicates punishment rather than anything substantial about the thing itself. To say precisely what pain is always raises the spectre of pains that don't fit the definition. Such exclusions (which have cropped up with an amazing frequency) reveal a politics of pain that has been central to the validation of painful experience for some, and has accounted for the invalidity of others. While contemporary medical science has found a barrage of novel ways to treat pain and to understand how pain works, new analgesic (from the Greek!) strategies and systems of knowledge still strive to account for the full implications of what it is like to be in pain. This is not, in the end, about semantics, but about experience. Linguistic heritage suggests that people have an implicit and comprehensive knowledge of pain in their own lives. Western medicine, for a large portion of its modern history, resisted quotidian experience, vernacular epistemology, and phenomenology (perhaps because they weren't expressed in these terms). It tended to work with narrow definitions, designed to fit mechanistic and dualistic understandings of the human. How this came to be, and how it is now changing, is the remarkable story of the history and experience of pain.

Chapter 2
Pain and piety

Pain and Christian practice

Ecce Homo: behold the man. These are the words associated with Pontius Pilate (d. 37 CE) upon presenting the bloodied, tortured, and pained body of Christ to the assembled masses, prior to crucifixion. The images associated with this scene became emblematic of virtuous suffering, and of the theological importance for Christians to endure bodily pain. The representation of Christ's *passion* in this moment has been preserved by the art world in the figure of the *vir dolorum*, or the man of pains, sometimes given as the 'man of sorrows' or the *Schmerzensmann*. Geergten tot Sint Jans (1465–95), the early Dutch school painter, produced a particularly fine *Man of Sorrows* (Figure 2), containing common theological inaccuracies. Christ is depicted surrounded by the instruments of his punishment, the whip and the birch, bleeding from the crown of thorns. He also wears the injury in his side given only after his crucifixion, also indicated by the puncture wounds in his hands. Curiously, given these post-crucifixion marks, Christ is found in the act of bearing the cross. But despite all this clear evidence of physical trauma, what does the facial expression painted by Geergten portray? It is not the clenched, narrow-eyed, paled figure of a man in bodily pain; it is the look of sorrow or grief; it depicts a hurt beyond the mere physical, echoed in the faces of the grieving witnesses and

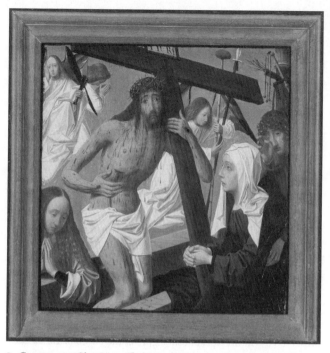

2. **Geertgen tot Sint Jans,** *Christus als Man van smarten* (*c.*1486).

angels who surround Christ. The wounds, the blood, the weapons are all figures that invite reflection on a suffering that goes beyond the mortification of flesh. A 21st-century viewer might readily recognize the expression of grief, but it does take extra work to understand the meaning and context of this grief.

Pain was a central pillar in Christian religious practice from the Roman world to the Counter Reformation of the 17th century, and arguably beyond. As Javier Moscoso and others have pointed out, pain was the foundation of medieval and early modern piety, as part of an ascetic quest to imitate the ultimate pain in Christ's passion. It was a pain not merely to be endured, but to be sought after, enhanced in any way imaginable, and, sometimes literally, sanctified. The imitation of the passion was celebrated in the lives of the Christian martyrs, whose placid countenances in the face of horrible tortures served as proof of the intervention of the saints, and, paradoxically, as evidence of their exaggerated resolve: a measure of unswerving faith and exemplary humanity. Meanwhile, such tortures informed medieval and early modern systems of justice and punishment. Long before pain came to be considered useful from an evolutionary point of view, pain was considered useful from moral, spiritual, and judicial points of view.

For Christians in medieval and early modern times, pain, suffering, and Christ's passion were defining features of life. The consequence of the Fall was that Eve's sorrow was multiplied, and that she would bring forth children in pain (*dolore* in the Latin Vulgate, *lupais* in the Greek Septuagint, *etzev* in Hebrew). Adam was cursed to labour in pain to take food from the earth. In both passages, Genesis 3:16 and 17, the concepts of labour (toil, or work) and pain are intermingled, as are grief and sorrow. Not for nothing is the process of giving birth called 'labour', which can be read as a direct synonym of pain. Sometimes vernacular translation fails to do justice to the semantic richness of the original terms, but it should be clear enough that the religious life, especially in medieval and early modern times, was dominated by the meaningful fact of being and coming to be in pain.

The long period of human history in which pain and suffering were actively sought by the pious as both evidence of their piety and as a (partial) guarantee of salvation is a challenge to the view that all pain is evil. Even the word 'piety' involves a linguistic entanglement of devotion and suffering. *Pieta*, most commonly associated with Mary's grieving over the dead body of Christ, and 'pity', which originally denoted a kind of suffering or compassion, are both etymologically associated with piety. Christ's spiritual suffering was betokened by a suffering of the flesh. To be like

Christ, the devoted sought ways to bring this kind of suffering unto themselves, mortifying the flesh in order to allow for the possibility of a communion with God at the level of the soul. There are many medieval and early modern accounts of *imitatio Christi* that demonstrate a kind of transcendence, where physical pain was indulged to the point that worldly considerations faded away, the focus being targeted precisely on the anguish of the soul and the affinity with Christ that this inward gaze brought about. While there were considerable changes and disagreements in the overarching value or end of imitating Christ's suffering, the notion of it being essentially useful was remarkably enduring.

In the pre-Reformed Catholic world, and even after in the Catholic centres of Europe, the extremity of Christ's physical suffering signified the extent of suffering at the level of the soul. The weight of this suffering symbolized the collective weight of humanity's sin. Such suffering proved difficult to represent. Those who wished to depict Christ's immaterial agonies had recourse only to the body and the facial expression to project an understanding of the ultimate pain. This often makes for a strange juxtaposition of facial placidity combined with an exaggerated corruption of the body. One of the most extraordinary examples, from the Holy Roman Empire and dating probably to the early 17th century (Figure 3), exemplifies a perceived need to make Christ's pain understood through graphic corporal disintegration. It emphasizes, through the calm, downturned face, that these injuries are only a figurative method for mere mortals to begin to grasp the weight of suffering on a spiritual level. Unlike many depictions of Christ on the cross, which include the spear wound to the side, inflicted to check that Christ was already dead, this carving is ambiguous about the moment it captures. There is no theological orthodoxy in depicting the limbs of Christ with flayed skin, exposed skeleton, and haemorrhaging blood from every part. This kind of construction of placidity in the face of extreme corporal punishment was typical of the depiction of the saints. Such punishments served also as a reference point for

18

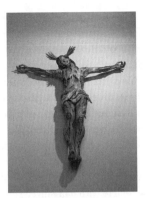

3. Christ on the Cross (17th century), Holy Roman Empire, from the Deutsches Historisches Museum.

the cruel and unusual treatment that awaited heretics, criminals, and witches.

Realizing images of the suffering Christ was not without theological difficulties. The obscure Gospel of Peter, of which fragments survive, points to the silence of Christ during crucifixion, 'as if in no pain', but this permits a contention that Christ's humanity was in question. If Christ was truly a human form, then his forbearance in the face of pain was a performance of great and virtuous self-control, or a mastery of mind and spirit over material afflictions. If there was really no pain inflicted through Christ's trial and crucifixion, then the virtuosity of resolve is lost.

No human pain could reach the extent of Christ's suffering on behalf of humanity, but to embrace pain after the fashion of Christ was to offset sin and therefore reduce the amount of suffering after death. In this sense, pain was considered by many to be a blessing, or an unmitigated good, since it promised a swifter route to redemption in the afterlife. It would have been heretical, given this view, to seek entirely to desensitize oneself to pain, though doubtless the pained sought remedies and often found them. But the virtuous and those of a particularly pious bent were to steel themselves to live with and through pain. Childbirth was as God intended. Painful disease was divinely inflicted. As Esther Cohen has pointed out in *The Modulated Scream*, this theological stance was the only way to resolve a tangible and all too readily observable ubiquity of suffering with the notion of an omnipresent Providence. Here we can account for the placid faces and stoical stories of the Christian martyrs, who met their fates with the conviction that gruesome punishment was only heightening the rewards that awaited them. Monastic orders embraced lives of ascetic hardship, replete with hair shirts, starvation, and flagellation (later it became *discipline*, a technical term denoting that the whip had migrated from the back to the buttocks) in order to prepare themselves for death and the afterlife. The fire of pain was to be welcomed for its perceived galvanizing and purifying qualities. The purified soul was closer to God.

Torture and punishment

The notion of pain as spiritually useful affords some insight into judicial practices of torture and punishment in Europe from the Roman to the early modern period that might otherwise seem strange and puzzling. Practices of torture were implicitly connected to theological understandings of pain insofar as pain was thought to purify sin and elicit truth. A judicial confession, just as with a spiritual confession, was thought to be reached through a process of painful experience. Whereas the latter was experienced as repentance, the former was evoked through torture. If pain was a way to the truth, the torturers of both presumed criminals and perceived heretics still had a problem. What if, wracked with every physical agony imaginable, the criminal maintained her innocence? What if the heretic refused to deny his God? Typically, the use of torture to get to the truth did not leave room for much a priori doubt about the guilt of the person in question. Yet the failure of torture, whether according to penal code or theology, to arouse the desired response to interrogation, threatened to undermine its whole rationale. The power of martyrology lay in the appropriation of a common knowledge about the power of pain to divine truth. If, in exquisite agony, the martyr neither renounced her belief nor denounced her God, then her convictions must have carried the weight of truth. The judicial power of torture to expose criminals was found to share this weakness.

If torture in advance of conviction was problematic, corporal punishment after conviction was no less so. From 1488, and for many centuries thereafter, Gerard David's (1460–1523) *Judgement of Cambyses* hung in the Town Hall at Bruges (Figure 4). Though it depicts an ancient scene, of the skinning alive of the corrupt judge Sisamnes in Persia, the figures in it sport contemporary dress and serve as a warning to magistrates to retain their integrity. Sisamnes' son, who replaced him as judge, sits on a throne bedecked in his father's skin, as a constant reminder. Sisamnes, restrained, grits his teeth. The flayers do their work with dispassionate attention. The onlookers show a remarkable calm, or else barely pay attention to the scene unfolding in front of them. What did it mean to witness such gruesome punishment? What did it mean even to behold such a painting of punishment, hanging in the space where justice was served?

There are countless European examples from the middle ages, but especially from the 16th century onwards, of corporal punishment as public spectacle. Pain was perhaps less of a personal corrective than a public warning, that a gruesome fate awaited those who transgressed the law. The trouble with the concept of public spectacle as horrific warning was that it depended on people freely turning up to watch. Public punishment, however awful to behold, was compelling, if not entertaining. But if the justification for corporal punishment spectacles was only loosely constructed, the justification for corporal punishment per se offered up a contradiction that risked undermining the theological discourse

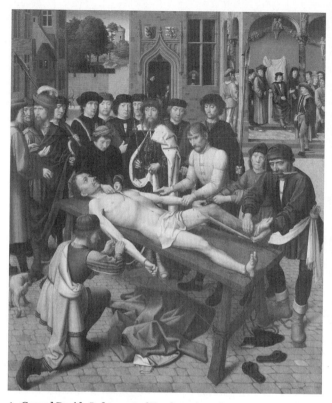

4. Gerard David, *Judgement of Cambyses* (1488).

that upheld the experience of pain as a Christian virtue. How could corporal punishment be exhibited as a fate to be avoided when, for many, it was precisely associated with the fate of martyrs who exemplified faith, piety, and virtue? One might justify corporal punishment in schools as an aid to learning—a practice that lasted hundreds of years—but administering pain as punishment to criminals was, by a Christian logic, to reward the condemned. As Enlightenment ideals began to supplant judicial retribution with penal reformation, so corporal punishment declined.

Patience as virtue

The virtuosity of sacred suffering gradually became less exclusively the province of martyrs and divines, and was widely appropriated. The accidentally afflicted in life—the ill, the injured, the infirm—began to see themselves as reaping the rewards of redeemed sin. The laity could connect their own pains to the suffering of Christ, invoking both a spirit of emulation and a reminder of the essentially sinful state of the human. If this brought the sufferer closer to God by analogy, the connection of pain to sin, and of sin to confession, personalized the relationship. Genuine remorse and repentance for sin was (supposed to be) experienced as an overwhelming physical and emotional pain, the sign of which was tears. Pain was the reward of a sinful nature, and a reflection on one's personal guilt heightened the pain of sin. A genuine personal acceptance of this guilt, coupled with repentance, was to move closer to God. As confessional practices among the laity expanded after the Fourth Lateran Council of 1215, the Catholic world in general became reconciled to the notion of the virtue of pain when coupled with repentance.

To say this is not to make the claim that people enjoyed their pains, illnesses, and suffering, but medicine until remarkably recently had little to offer by way of remedying the feeling of pain, if it was interested in so doing. The 'patient'—literally, the sufferer—was left to dwell on the rewards to be wrought by and through pain. Not for nothing do people say 'patience is a virtue'. Moreover, the inescapability of pain of all sorts, right up until the 19th century, was hardly something to be dealt with in private, as if it were some personal affliction. In Europe, at least, people lived in a world of pain, of shared understandings of suffering, and of a shared understanding of the purpose of hurt. Even when people sought remedy for their pains, which they undoubtedly did, they did so in the knowledge that their pain had a value—held in common—beyond mere suffering. Pain was not merely noxious;

it was a means to an (improved) end. After the Reformation, pain remained an important sign of God's love among Protestants, even if no amount of it could wipe away the stain of sin. Protestants still tended to think that the joyous embrace of suffering among the martyrs was virtuous, since being afflicted with pain not only called to mind the righteous sufferings of Christ, but also might have been a sign of being among the elect. When in pain, the good Protestant could use it to channel his faith, though it had no effect on his sin. There was, however, no longer any need to seek out this suffering, to flagellate or discipline, nor any Stoic obligation to conquer pain as if it were not there.

Attaching a positive purpose to pain was not limited to Christian traditions. In *The Ascetic Self* (2004), Gavin Flood notes that the willing acceptance of pain as a 'method for the body's transcendence' is 'a common feature of ascetic tradition'. Specific practices are diverse. Tantric ascetics in medieval Kashmir, for example, following Shaivist theology, sought a state of transcendent subjectivity by putting themselves in physical pain and concentrating exclusively on this pain. In Hindu thought more generally, suffering is thought to be caused by desires of which the sufferer may not be consciously aware. To alleviate the misery of pain requires the sufferer to identify the desire and remove it.

In Buddhism, meanwhile, pain is considered to be implicit in human existence, understood as what Lih-Mik Chen and others describe as a 'physical-emotional-mental-spiritual complex that defines the nature of human experience'. The Buddhist transcendental ideal involves not the elimination of pain, but rather a process of becoming emotionally detached from it by following the 'right paths'. The inescapability of pain in this tradition makes it a form of meaningful living and thinking, placing it at the centre of efforts to abstain from desire, which in turn fortifies the body and cleanses the soul. Pain is similarly central to Confucian cosmology in China, an individual's pain being the primary indicator of human sensitivity and therefore a clue to the sufferings of others. To be without pain, or without the capacity to suffer it, is to lose one's humanity.

A theological problem

In modern times, pain has remained an important theological problem. With an increase in secular and atheistic dissent in public discourse, centuries of theological musing on the subject of pain, seeking to reconcile the existence of suffering with an all-powerful benevolent deity, have frequently been questioned. The classic observation, often recalled, is that of Charles Darwin (1809–82), who observed the breeding habits of the Ichneumon wasp. It injects its eggs into a host insect without killing it. The host unwittingly incubates the eggs, and then provides the first meal for the new larvae when they hatch, eating their host from the inside out. How could a benevolent God countenance such horror, such torture, such painful cruelty? Of course, such an account of pain and cruelty would have been meaningless before modernity had extended the compass of pain and suffering to the non-human world. But even if such gruesome exemplars from nature are not persuasive, contemporary commentators often point to the surfeit of human suffering that persists without succour, all of our medicinal and anaesthetic advancements notwithstanding.

C.S. Lewis (1898–1963), writing in the theatre of the Second World War, when pain and suffering abounded with renewed ardour, made a concerted effort again to reconcile the world of pain with a loving God. The blame for human suffering, he averred, belonged to humanity, and had done so since the Fall. If humans suffer it is because they are faulty. The actions of a loving God cause people pain, because through His love He tries to improve people, to mould them, to *discipline* them into a better form. In *The Problem of Pain* (1940), Lewis remarks: 'God…shouts in our pains: it is His megaphone to rouse a dead world'. To ask for less of such suffering, according to Lewis, is to ask for less of God's love, not more. It is difficult to see much lasting traction for this argument among cultures formed in the Judeo-Christian tradition. The notion of martyrdom has survived elsewhere, but hardly in the mode of a life redeemed through suffering. Hundreds of years of pain conceived of as a virtue have been steadily eroded by the forces of secularization, utilitarianism, mechanism, and medicine. It is to the mechanistic view that we now turn, the advent of which saw the concept of what pain materially is, and to whom (or what) it can apply, completely overhauled.

Chapter 3
Pain and the machine

If vernacular understandings of pain have continuously stated the entanglement of body and mind (or soul), physical and emotional, from where came the notion of mind-body dualism that dominated Western medicine from the Enlightenment? The impact of that dualistic approach will be dealt with later, but first it is necessary to establish the architecture of dualism with reference to pain. And although this account will begin with the Enlightenment philosopher René Descartes (1596–1650), the blame should probably not be laid at his feet (or, at least, not directly).

Descartes and the machine

Descartes famously reduced the functioning of bodies to mechanics. Animals were like intricate clocks, mere unfeeling machines. The human distinction lay in the possession of a rational soul, which inhabited the machine like a pilot. What happened to the human body called the attention of the human soul, which moved with the machine without reducing to it. The thinking 'I' of Descartes' machine, an immaterial soul of divine origin, led the readers of Descartes to debate the import of a separation of mind and matter. But Descartes, at least as far as the human was concerned, forcefully asserted the separation in a complex way, rather than the simplistic concept that has been so

27

often attributed to him. Certainly, if the question is of animal pain, then the debate about whether non-human beings can suffer *at all* is attributable to him. Descartes' human, however, was not a separable entity of body and soul, so long as the body was alive, but a monistic union of body-mind or body-soul, which could not be reduced to its components.

True, in his *Meditations* (1641), Descartes insisted that the thinking thing (*res cogitans*) did not depend on a body, but when Descartes' body was affected by pain, *he* felt it; that is, at the level of the rational soul there was a disturbance (of thought), caused by the disruption or injury of the body with which the soul was conjoined. He talked of an 'admixture' (*permixtione*) of mind and body when it came to the senses (e.g. hunger or pain). The human body in pain was not merely a reflex mechanism akin to a bell on the end of a rope, but a body-mind that only *felt* pain because the mind was inseparable from its corporeal seat. If it were otherwise, according to Descartes, the human thinking thing would look upon bodily injury (lesion) as the pilot of a vessel would look upon a damaged boat. Clearly, as Descartes searched himself for answers, the human appreciation of pain was not simply one of pure understanding, but one of inherent involvement with bodily stuff.

So why the confusion? After Descartes' death, editions of his *Treatise on Man* (1662) were issued with illustrations, including what is probably the most commonly reproduced image of the pain mechanism. Search the internet for 'Descartes Pain' and you'll find the image of a man kneeling with his foot next to a small fire repeated endlessly (Figure 5). The depiction of the pain pathway—the mechanism for a pain reflex exactly like the aforementioned bell pull—has been repeatedly re-cast in words to sum up Descartes' thinking on how pain worked, largely ignoring his fuller account in the *Meditations*. The image has been copied and adapted to the point of becoming folk expertise. Patrick Wall (1925–2001), who perhaps did more than anyone to try to break

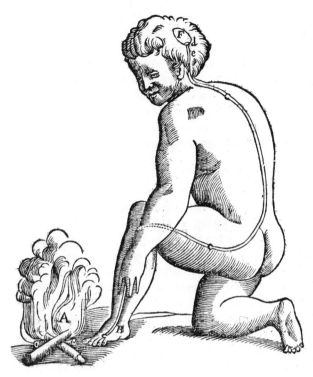

5. The Pain Pathway, from René Descartes, *Traite de l'homme* (1664).

the mind-body dualistic approach to pain in the late 20th century, despised the image and what it stood for, not least because it didn't say a great deal about most pain for most people. Pain, by this representation, is reducible to the sequence injury→pain→movement, in that order.

The reach of the simplistic reduction of Descartes' understanding of pain went far further than his more complex grappling with the relationship of the mind in a body. One significant community of sufferers, if that is indeed a suitable description, which has been most affected by so-called Cartesian thinking has been the world of non-human animals. In this respect at least, Descartes directly aided an enduring impression that animals, lacking an immortal soul and lacking reason, were mere machines without the capacity to feel pain. In what is perhaps his best-known work, *The Discourse on Method* (1637), animals were described as being like clocks, comprised of incomparable wheels and springs by virtue of their divine Designer. Any outward appearance of suffering was a mere consequence of mechanical operations in the animal, no different to that in an automaton.

Animal pain

The idea that animals suffer exquisite pain has existed since the time of Plutarch (45–120 CE), but did not extend beyond a few intellectuals until the 1960s. Even though Descartes' 'clockwork' analogy for the animal machine did not reach too far within the English-speaking world, its influence was nevertheless felt and co-mingled with a widespread notion (still official doctrine in the Catholic church) that animals did not possess a rational soul. Not only were they incapable of rationally conceiving—emotionally processing—suffering, torment, and the fears that coalesce around pain, but their existence was entirely material, mortal, and finite. In a context where the meaning of pain was inextricably bound up with the status of the immortal soul and what might happen to it in the afterlife, the pain of an animal (if any were acknowledged) was meaningless. In such a cosmology, one could no more be cruel to an animal as to a clod of earth. When this was superadded to the doctrine of human dominion over the beasts, as in the Christian tradition, then any scruples about using animals for entertainment, work, or experiment melted away, at least as far as the moral status of the animal was concerned.

Surprisingly, perhaps, such views survived into the Utilitarian age, where a balance-sheet of pleasure and pain determined the moral status of every action. The father of Utilitarianism in the late 18th century, Jeremy Bentham (1748–1832), pursued a theory of maximizing pleasure and minimizing pain to its ultimate ends. To kill a living thing was, from a strictly Utilitarian point of view, a favourable act, for in Bentham's opinion an animal would suffer all the more if left to live and would be none the worse for being dead. Death was a merciful end to suffering, which defined life in a natural state. The moral problem, therefore, was how to continue to condemn the killing of another human. For Bentham, the only difference between killing a man and killing an animal was that murder, by example, inspired fear in the hearts of other men, thereby adding to the degree of aggregate suffering among the human population. Since he saw no capacity for the spread of fear among animals, there was a clear categorical and ethical difference in putting them to the sword. It should not be lost upon us, however, that Bentham saw nothing intrinsically wrong with the killing of a man apart from this terrible example of fear. It was *humanity*, in both senses of the word, that was to keep us from harming each other.

Descartes' view, then, coloured the rationalist science of the Enlightenment, justified the new attempts to conquer nature, emboldened men (typically) to assert their superiority, and ushered in an unapologetic rise of experimentalism in which animals were the chief objects of study. Animals would become central to understanding the mechanics of pain, since they served as soulless analogues of human machines. Even where Descartes' reach was relatively limited, as in England, an apparent ubiquity of animal pain at human hands was readily justified in the name of increases in knowledge. This became especially apparent from the middle of the 19th century, when a thirst for knowledge about human physiology seemed to depend on a degree of animal pain in the experimental laboratory.

Victorian hand-wringing about the amount of animal pain in the world was mollified in part by the thought that some of this pain would usher in a profound diminution of pain for both humans and animals in the future. Animal pain in the laboratory, if it existed, could be instrumental—it could be used as negative means for positive ends. These outcomes comprised an imagined future of improved surgical techniques; clinical advances in the prevention and treatment of injury and disease, based on an improved understanding of animal bodies and pathogens; and the development of new drugs. Nineteenth-century physiologists answered those who worried about a rising tide of animal 'victims' by reference to the mechanical nature of animal bodies. Anaesthetized animals, incapable of feeling any pain, were made to 'dance' and grimace by the application of electrical stimulation. Muscle tissue could be completely isolated from its original animal and still have its reflex actions stimulated by specially designed machines. James Crichton-Browne (1840–1938), famous Victorian neurologist and medical psychologist, decried those who protested about the writhings of agony and painful grimaces of monkeys whose brains had effectively already been destroyed. These critics were fooled by appearances. Such signs were no more indications of pain than the 'screams' of a piano when its keys were struck. Descartes' imagery was highly persuasive, especially to those whose work depended on animal experimentation.

Pain knowledge

It was a chemical innovation that allowed the Cartesian denial of animal pain to finally give way. This was not to the benefit of animal lives, necessarily. The advent of surgical anaesthesia radically altered both the nature of surgery on humans and the ethical debate about animal experimentation. The properties of ether had been discovered in 1846 in Boston by William T.G. Morton (1819–68); those of chloroform had been discovered by James Young Simpson (1811–70) in Edinburgh the following year. A debate about the ethics of administering anaesthetics to humans emerged immediately, and it took time before the practice was widely employed. Women, in particular, faced resistance to pain-free childbirth because of the adherence to those doctrines that stressed the divine intention of painful labour. As for animals, physiologists and their supporters argued that safeguarding against pain put all experiments within ethical bounds. The capacity of animals to suffer was conclusively acknowledged only once the capacity to anaesthetize them had been established.

Yet the heyday of animal experimentation from the 1870s to the First World War, with the constant background noise about the question of pain, served to give rise to experiments designed precisely to measure pain. The emergence of a professional faith in mechanical objectivity—that is, the belief that nature should speak for itself without the subjective idealizing interpretation of the scientist—led to a number of devices designed to read and quantify pain. It was thought that machines could be designed better to measure animal (including human) experience. Just as blood pressure, blood chemistry, pulse, and so on could be charted by machines, so, it was hoped, could pain. The rapid spread of Charles Darwin's notion that all animals were fundamentally connected and therefore physiologically alike led to the acceptance of animals—from frogs to dogs—being used in physiological experiments as human analogues. Darwin himself was perhaps the most prominent figure in the period to argue for the virtues of physiological experimentation, under anaesthesia where possible, but even without it if experimentation could add to the store of human knowledge. Knowledge of animal pain would unlock the mysteries of human pain. Having tacitly acknowledged that animals suffered pain by agreeing to administer anaesthetics to them, the world of physiology set about understanding the mechanics of pain, which inevitably involved withholding those anaesthetics. This was a re-capitulation of the Cartesian view, but with the rather more useful experimental conclusion that animal pain was not different in kind to human pain. Physiologists, recognizing that pain was an unpleasant experience in humans and animals alike, nevertheless set out to find the 'wheels and springs' that made it work.

Central to the mechanical interest in both the measurement and the functioning of pain was the notion that pain was purely physical. The animal analogues that stood in for humans during pain-research experiments helped to cement the separation of mind and body, emotional and physical pain. For even if Darwinism had ensured that animal physiology could be used as a viable model for human physiology, the rise from the end of the 19th century of behaviourism ensured that any budding signs of emotional continuity between animals and humans were cut off. Up until that point, early work in the new field of comparative psychology had pursued the logical implications of the Darwinian project, asserting that just as differences among animal bodies were differences of degree and not differences in kind, such was the same among animal minds. Some even tried to develop a monistic version of Darwinian evolution, where minds and bodies were seen essentially to be intrinsically intertwined and mutually co-dependent parts of functioning wholes.

This changed with the 1894 statement of British psychologist Conwy Lloyd Morgan's (1852–1936) 'canon', which destroyed the rationale for investigating animal emotions. Its axiom was as follows: 'In no case is an animal activity to be interpreted in terms of higher psychological processes if it can be fairly interpreted in terms of processes which stand lower in the scale of psychological evolution and development'. In other words, if expressions that looked like emotional feeling or communication could possibly be explained by reflex action, physiological structure, or mechanical operations, then such explanations should be considered the most likely. Behaviourism's nemesis was anthropomorphism, in particular the projection of human emotional characteristics onto other animals. Of course, the contiguous lines of evolutionary trees ought to have implied some such projection, tempered by cognitive and other abilities, but behaviourism did not entertain subjective experience as analytically useful. Behaviourism essentially re-asserted a Cartesian mechanistic worldview.

In the process, pain research became trapped in the mind-body dualism that behaviourism favoured.

Measuring pain

The mechanisms designed to test for pain in humans in the first half of the 20th century were strongly associated with the need to measure what constituted pain from a purely physical point of view. Subjective qualities or, more simply, evidence from the person being measured, were overlooked at best and consciously discounted at worst. Pain levels should be objectively measurable, or so went the rationale; how a person felt about her pain was a matter of character, morals, even gender or race. Coupled with the enduring idea that the primary function of medicine was to detect injury and disease and hopefully to cure them, pain was of secondary interest only as an indicator as to where the 'real' problem lay. Pain measurement and pain objectivity were therefore purposefully distant, cool, not so much lacking in compassionate rationale as being outside the realm of compassion altogether.

What researchers were looking for, primarily, was an index of pain sensitivity. They wanted to find the point at which pain was detectable in humans. It was thought that, under controlled conditions, this would clearly indicate the degree of civilization, criminal tendencies, or relative 'savagery' of a subject. Pain thresholds—the points at which pain is considered to be unbearable—had long been known to vary, but it was important to find out if there were fundamental differences in the extent to which pain could be felt at all. The modern history of pain was built upon research that asserted that certain 'types' of people were either more sensitive to painful stimuli or less able to bear it. This had profound practical consequences for suffering patients who sought the help of professional medicine. The level of treatment—the extent to which analgesics were administered and compassionate care was offered—could be directly correlated with race, age, and gender.

To manufacture devices—algometers or dolorimeters—that could measure pain sensitivity was, uncannily enough, the province of psychologists as well as physiologists. Cesare Lombroso (1835–1909), famous for his categorization of the criminal type in his book *L'uomo delinquente* ('The Criminal Man', 1876), adopted a device devised by German physiologist Emil du Bois-Reymond (1818–1896) that measured both the sensitivity and the pain threshold of individuals with an electrical stimulus. Pain in the criminal type, he concluded, was 'much less acute and sometimes non-existent'. Proof could be read off the pain scale (Figure 6). Lombroso's research was based on a theory that criminality was heritable and that the signs of it were physical. He set about proving it by comparing the characteristics of criminals, dead and alive, with non-criminals. The results were fantastic, highly

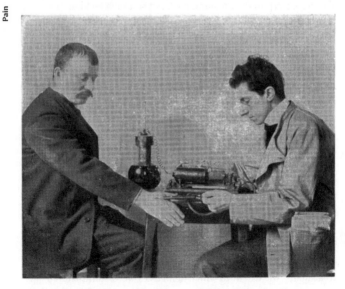

6. Algometer, from Cesare Lombroso, *Criminal Man* (1911).

influential, and baseless. His example, however, is indicative of wider trends. The mechanistic thrust of algometric investigations took psychologists away from speculations about the immaterial workings of the mind to the material and concretely measurable sensitivity of the skin, and with it to the processing capacities of the brain (as distinct from the mind).

Another programme, in 1940, used the heat from a lamp, concentrated on an area of the skin, to chart the temperature at which patients at the New York Hospital felt heat to be painful, and again to chart the temperature at which the pain became unbearable. It was a renewed attempt to make pain an objective, measurable quality, with two implications. First, if pain could be accurately measured perhaps it could be more effectively treated. And, second, if pain was measurable then patient reactions to pain could be better assessed, or dismissed. Having a mechanical readout of pain would allow the clinician to go beyond, or even eliminate entirely, the subjective element of pain, with all its metaphors and imprecision. The perceived tendency of some to over-report and others to under-report their degree of suffering would have no bearing on the administration of pain medication. The trouble was, it didn't work. Or at least, the results weren't repeatable from one laboratory to another, since test subjects could be disciplined to tolerate variable levels of pain. At the very least, a common range of values might be found for when the stimulus was first sensed under controlled conditions, but pain thresholds were shown to vary widely and for a whole host of reasons, not least that individuals are rarely, if ever, in 'neutral' states.

Mechanical theories

If mechanical pain research owed much to Descartes, it was because he was thought to have said something so demonstrably obvious that it only remained to discover the specific mechanisms by which a 'pain pathway' worked. Following Descartes, the human machine was presumed to include a specific pain system, joining nerve endings in the skin to the spinal cord and to a 'pain centre' in the brain. With great industry, physiologists from the mid-19th century onwards started to look for specific pain receptor nerves, or 'nociceptors'. All manner of human qualities and experiences were thought to be measurable and quantifiable. Brains were weighed to establish a racial and gendered order of intellect. Skulls were measured to demonstrate degrees of civilization. Faces were photographed in ingenious ways in order to depict the 'criminal classes'. And 'pain fibres' were described as being particularly involved in this or that type of pain, or this or that magnitude of pain. The brain, according to this approach, was a mere receiver of specific pain inputs. The basic premise, that a pain scale could be correlated to injury intensity, has been, since the 1960s, convincingly demonstrated to be false.

What has survived this mechanical reduction to be refined by contemporary neuroscience is the sorting out of different nerve endings according to what kind and what degree of stimulus makes them fire. We now know that there is no absolute correlation of experience and nerve stimulation. We still talk of 'nociceptors', but what they signal has to be interpreted by the brain before it becomes pain. The other problem with mechanical simplicity is that while it seemed adequately to describe what happened when a man's foot entered the fire, it could not account for pains that seemed to endure beyond the confines of specific nerve damage or direct stimulation. More advanced mechanical explanations were put forward to try to resolve this mystery.

Various 'pattern' theories emerged between the 1880s and the 1950s to account for pain responses that seemed to be out of proportion to initial nerve stimulation. It was assumed that some process had to be happening in the spinal cord, sparked by the original peripheral stimulus, which was self-sustaining or even self-enhancing. As nervous-system mechanics increasingly employed the metaphorical language of electrical engineering (something it retains to a large degree), so one could begin to imagine 'feedback loops' of neurons within the 'wiring' of the spinal cord, which 'reverberate' and excite neighbouring neurons. As the image implies, such a pattern of nervous activation could be kept up in perpetuity, irrespective of the healing or even disappearance of the initial cause (hence phantom limb pain, for example). The problem with this vision was that electrical circuit boards with feedback loops are easier to imagine than to discover. Similarly, pain pathologies have been imagined as the failure of 'normal' pain 'circuitry', with the result being the equivalent of a signal boost in certain types of pain fibre. Elements of each of these theories have proved useful in the construction of more holistic theories of pain experience in contemporary neuroscience and pain management, but they have had to go beyond a purely mechanical relation of stimulus to experience.

Only from the 1960s did criticism begin to emerge from within and without scientific establishments—notably by Thomas Kuhn (1922–96) and, later, by Bruno Latour (b. 1947)—pointing to the important influence of social context in the making of scientific work and its driving ideas and assumptions. More recently, Lorraine Daston and Peter Galison re-cast objectivity itself as an affect in their book *Objectivity* (2007). Facts are now considered by many to be always framed, constructed, partial. Uncertainty opened up new avenues of research, but change emerged slowly. As early as 1894, the American psychologist Henry Rutgers Marshall (1852–1927) had argued forcefully that both pleasure and pain were differential qualities of mental states; they were 'elements of consciousness', tied to emotions, to the senses, to the mind, and to the body, but such holistic thinking held little sway in the same year that saw the birth of behaviourism with Morgan's canon. When pain research did open up to the possibility of emotional and social components of pain in the 1970s, the limitations imposed by a perceived need to make definitive measurements, judgements, and diagnoses within medical practice kept the mechanical relation between pain and injury alive.

The imagery of harm

Doctors in the clinical environment have been working with a multidimensional understanding of pain for many decades. The McGill Pain Questionnaire was developed by Ronald Melzack (b. 1929) and Warren Torgerson (1924–99) in 1971. It was the first elaborate medical assessment technique for the quality of a person's pain experience to put control in the hands of the patient herself. The pain questionnaire grouped adjectives and metaphors of pain into categories of intensity and then divided the categories along the lines of sensation, affect, evaluation, and miscellaneous, combining these with a diagrammatic location of the pain on a representation of the body and a general appraisal of other symptoms and general lifestyle. The premise, confirmed in many cases, was that certain pain syndromes were described by sufferers in similar terms. The qualitative insights from the pain questionnaire would therefore allow the clinician a better chance of a correct diagnosis in the first instance, based on the patient's own evaluation of her pain.

While this seems, at first glance, to have been a successful response to the re-introduction of affective qualities of pain experience and a new direction in clinical appraisal, there were limitations. The pain questionnaire, translated into many languages, made use of the common weapon trope, or the metaphor of being wounded, sliced, stabbed, shot, pounded, or crushed. A number of scholars have pointed out the remarkable endurance of this kind of metaphor for describing human pain experiences. It is as if there is no literal way of giving utterance to pain, and that these images of harm are all we have to turn to. But the apparent limitation belies an astounding richness and depth of description. Over time, of course, weapons change along with the imaginative and figurative ways of describing what weapons do to people. Moreover, as one moves from one language to another, one finds nuance of expression, meaning, and context that defies easy universalizing categorization. The politics of translation, let alone the methods, always raise the question of whose words are forming the fundamental categories: those of the patients, the doctors, or the translators?

Once language is acknowledged as a significant bearer of information about a person's subjective experience, it is difficult then to confine it to prescribed definitions and categories. The pain questionnaire did a good job in collating the common pain descriptors of the time, in English, but it also risked determining pain descriptors for the future. Handing a patient a list of descriptors and asking him to 'fit' his pain to them might be considered a highly suggestive and influential strategy, based on the assumption that these words in particular capture the essence of pain. While they may work for some, others will have to strive to match what they feel to what is listed, even though it doesn't feel right. Others still will wonder about the veracity of their pain if it doesn't seem to fit at all. Attempts to fix a linguistic scheme in order to hear the subjectivity of pain had the effect of objectivizing it.

Ultimately, the affective qualities of pain being searched for in the 1970s and 1980s were fitted into regulated schema of fixed values, just as physical pain values had been subjected to mechanical objectivity. Patients' voices were heard, but also pre-empted. According to a study by Ann Harrison, when the McGill Pain Questionnaire was translated into Arabic in Kuwait, the compilers were well aware of the linguistic slippages, even among a localized community. Educated Kuwaitis likely knew English, had larger vocabularies, and described their pain in words 'too esoteric for the average patient to understand'. Did that mean their pain experiences were also different? We shall likely never know because their input was consciously avoided. Curiously, the Arabic translators also avoided the help of chronic-pain patients because 'their pain ratings differ systematically from those … experiencing acute pain'. When one remembers that the McGill Pain Questionnaire was originally devised to try to get inside the pain experience of pain syndromes—that is, it is aimed precisely at chronic-pain sufferers—then one must conclude that the act of translation had also obscured the conceptual purpose of the tool. Twentieth-century medicine's need for value-neutral objects of inquiry was an obstacle to exploring a core component of pain experience since that core component was, itself, a subjective value, an affect. Linguistic representations of pain affect—what people say when they say how they feel—defy the rigours of tabulation and categorization. The translators in Kuwait experienced this first hand, finding that words classified as 'sensory' in the original English were, when translated, better fitted in the 'affective' or 'evaluative' categories. 'There is good reason to suppose,' the authors concluded, 'that pain categories may vary from culture to culture'. They couldn't find a translation for 'shooting' pain. Meanwhile, the Italian translation for 'shooting' offered up a pain 'like the rebound of a bed spring'. In all, the McGill Pain Questionnaire was translated into twenty-six languages, according to a 2009 study from the George Institute for International Health in Sydney. That study found that testing of the effectiveness of these translations was generally poor, and the use of 'non-English versions' should be 'undertaken with caution'. Different versions of the questionnaire contained between 42 and 176 pain descriptors. Such is the richness of human utterances of pain experiences. That they resist or defy categorical tabulation only demonstrates that people are not, or not entirely, machines.

Chapter 4
Pain and civilization

It has been well documented that, with the demise of Catholic practices of mortification, the moral virtue of pain was replaced, in 18th-century Europe, with the opposite notion that by no means was pain necessary for salvation, or even as an indication of moral virtuosity. On the contrary, pleasure emerged as the principle of the virtuous, with a turning away from pain as a personal and social evil. At the same time, the 18th century saw the dawn of the 'age of sensibility', in which heightened practices of civility and urbanity seemed to bring with them a more acute capacity for suffering, both physically and emotionally. As the Utilitarian era dawned, which defined the Good according to an aggregate of pleasure and happiness, it seemed that the most civilized members of society were all the more likely to succumb to the pains of civilization. Here enters the quotidian language of nerves and the nervous, the rise of the modern hysteric, and thereafter the neurasthenic, neuralgic, and shell-shocked. Pain in the modern period became a problem not because there was suddenly more of it, but because it became apparently pointless. No moral end was served by it. In sweeping away the moral purpose of pain, there was a correlative increase in anxiety about coming to be in pain.

Pain politics

Pain has never been entirely the province of the sufferer. Intellectuals, philosophers, doctors, nurses, and legislators have had a disproportionate stake in saying what it is, who has it (and who doesn't), and what should be done about it. In short, pain has been defined, delimited, and determined by a legion of people not so much in pain as in power. The 18th-century preoccupation with 'civilization' was not only defined by cultural, intellectual, and economic markers, but also by sensory and experiential distinctions. Those who self-identified as living within civilization were compelled to try to understand what set them apart as humans. This was a highly gendered, highly racialized, and distinctly classed process of establishing a framework for inclusion and exclusion. Humanness itself seemed to be measurable, with civilized men being the most human, and 'savages', working-class people, and also women and children, being among the least. The distance to animality among some configurations of human being was narrowed to a small mark of distinction. For those identified as female 'savages' or female children, the distance to a bare animal existence was practically nothing.

A major distinguishing marker of these gradations of humanity was the capacity to feel pain, or degree of sensitivity to pain. The schema of pain sensitivity might seem absurd on first reading, but we live with the legacy of this ordering. The politics of pain still affect the treatment people tend to receive when they complain of pain in clinical settings. In order to make sense of some of the remarkable historical categorizations of pain sensitivity, it is helpful to look at the ways in which this still happens today. A number of studies from across Europe and North America have found, repeatedly, that women report their pain to a greater extent than men. The mode of their reporting is also marked by affective behaviour that is stereotypically ascribed to women: tears, emotionality, etc. Men, on the other hand, are thought to under-report their pain, as part of a perception of the unmanliness of complaint and of pain tolerance or forbearance as a masculine quality. The clinical results of this gendered behaviour, which is not reducible to biological or genetic differences in the vast majority of cases, but which is learned behaviour within certain cultural environments, are significant. The assumption that women over-report is coupled with a tendency to under-treat, under-medicate, and take them less seriously in their expressions of pain. Conversely, men, assumed to under-report, are given more attention and, to a corresponding degree, more narcotics for their pain. A direct causal connection between gendered behaviour (and experience) and variable administration of analgesics is difficult to establish. The relationship is, however, highly correlated.

These gendered behaviours are learned in childhood. Very young infants do not demonstrably differ along sex lines in their manifestations of pain. Despite knowledge that these culturally inscribed differences do affect how pain is experienced—what people report probably does bear on how they feel—the treatment of pain in medical settings has tended to imply that there is a pain reality below the surface and beyond the superficial indications uttered by the patient. This adherence to a sort of 'pain standard' endures in practice, even though many studies, such as that by Carly Miller and Sarah Newton on 'Pain Perception and Expression', have confirmed that best practice should follow the maxim, 'Pain is whatever the experiencing person says it is, existing whenever he or she says it does'.

Birth and infant pain

This particular iteration of a 'pain standard' is by no means a timeless one. The shifting rhetorical constructions of civilization have set the standard at many different and often wholly contradictory levels. Across the history of modernity, as Joanna Bourke has shown in *The Story of Pain* (2014), children were assumed to be both less and more sensitive to pain. By far the more damaging in the annals of the history of childhood has been the former, which peaked from the late 19th century and endured until at least the 1980s. All manner of agents, from doctors and surgeons to priests, philosophers, and scientists, claimed that babies—being barely sentient—were wholly or partially insensitive to pain. Injury, surgery, and illness could, therefore, be passed over without due concern. These conclusions were reached through historical understandings of how to gauge painful experience in another. Since reason was so inherently tied to speech, a being that could not speak its pain was assumed not to be able feel pain at all (the same went for animals). Enlightenment thinkers even questioned whether human infants had an immortal soul at birth, or whether this emerged later with the onset of a clearly identifiable sentience. No immortal soul: no pain. Even though such discussions have long since become arcane, the notion that babies don't have a particularly acute sensitivity to pain endured well into the 20th century. Lack of complete brain or nervous-system development, coupled with concerns about the administration of opiates in babies, led to a general conclusion that it was safer to assume that infants felt no pain. In any case, if they did, it was assumed they would carry no lasting memory of it and be none the worse for it.

While babies certainly do suffer pain, there is no clear way to establish the exact nature of it. Some psychologists who maintain a universalist position have tried to demonstrate the similarity between the pained facial expressions of infants and mice, among other animals. There is widespread evidence, as presented by Martin Schiavenato and others, of a 'common and universal expression' of pain that is 'hardwired and present at birth'. This facial expression, however, may only tell us of the presence of pain and not about its experience. We do not know, because we cannot directly access how the infant feels, what the experience is like. Parents comforting the infant whose ears hurt as an aeroplane ascends or descends know that the experience is painful, but also that the child's suffering is based on a lack of understanding of what is happening, why, and how to remedy it. As adults, we can only imagine what it would be like not to understand. We stretch our sympathies, but we are ontologically bound by experience. Doubtless, there is significant emotional involvement in the child; but what will later be articulated as 'fear', or as 'anger', or as 'anxiety' remain inarticulate in the infant. What we can say with certainty is that children subjected to pain in early life are likely to suffer long-term consequences, including changes in the central nervous system and changes in the biological stress response in adulthood. In short, infants who undergo painful interventions in the early stages of life are *made* more susceptible to pain, considered as a holistic experience involving mind, body, and society. It is highly likely, according to Gale Page, an expert on the 'biobehavioural' effects of pain experiences in infancy, that pained infants grow into adults who have heightened avoidance behaviour and 'social hypervigilance', and whose pain sensitivity is correspondingly higher. Clearly, the inchoate fears of infancy are deeply involved with, and have a lasting effect on, the experience of pain.

If pain in babies has been the source of confusion in the setting of the 'pain standard', the means of their arrival has long bewildered doctors. The history of 'modern' and 'civilized' society is marked by the increase of medical intervention in childbirth. The history of recorded knowledge about childbirth has largely excluded insights from women themselves. Since the institutions of both learning and medicine have been the provinces of men only for most of their history, the best first-hand sources of what it is like to give birth were neglected until remarkably recently. With the drift of Western childbirth away from home and into clinical settings from the late 19th century, so women themselves became alienated from a community of shared experience and colloquial knowledge, heightening fears and anxieties about parturition.

Giving birth has always been *laborious*, and certainly dangerous, but an increase in fear corresponding to uncertainty can be correlated with a heightened experience of pain. Here the idea of pain as necessarily something unpleasant might mislead us into thinking that the most fundamental act in the continued existence of humans must be, and have always been, *terrible*. Many women today do not recognize this as an accurate description of what happens to them in childbirth. Doubtless, there has always been pain, and doubtless it was often unpleasant, but a context of community knowledge, reassurance, and experience helped diminish fear and therefore affected the quality of pain. Terror became more acute in part through the disempowerment of women who lost agency and control over birth. Through the 18th century and into the 19th, women's accounts of their own anticipation of childbirth relate more frequent fears and more complete assignation of responsibility to medical agents.

The gradual re-classification of childbirth from a natural procedure to a medical one was the slow encroachment of the institutions of medicine into women's autonomy over their own bodies. This was the result of women themselves having become isolated from discourses, cultures, and communities of 'natural' birthing. The result has undeniably been a reduction in both infant and mother mortality, but it is questionable whether the 20th-century history of 'civilized' childbirth contained either less pain or more pleasure. Birthing options today in many countries have returned a measure of contextual control to women, empowering them with both knowledge and reassurance to limit birth trauma and fear.

Race

Perceptions of racial difference have had an equally marked effect on both the experience and treatment of pain, as pain became the sole province of medicine through the 19th century. Received opinion among 19th-century 'civilized' opinion makers was that 'primitive' women gave birth without much pain or discomfort, partly because their physical racial differences made them less sensitive, in accord with their 'natural', animal-like existence. Civilization itself came bundled with more pain, since it was in part defined by heightened sensitivity and a closeness to emotional upheaval. While a recent attempt by Zatzick and Dimsdale to nail down substantial differences among diverse 'races' found no discernible variation in controlled tests, there are nevertheless strong prevailing cultural currents that stratify pain sensitivity and pain threshold according to crude delineations of human types. Just as with the question of age, perceptions of pain sensitivity among various 'races' have changed over time. In the natural philosophy of the 18th century, through the birth of anthropology and evolutionary biology in the 19th, African 'types', for example, were considered to be basically insensitive to pain. However, a more recent study based at the University of Florida found African Americans to be much more sensitive to pain than people with 'European' ancestry. The second half of the 20th century saw a protracted contest among American scholars with different disciplinary and ideological motives to map pain according to racial origins, with Jews in particular being marked out as more sensitive to pain. Basic pain schemes reinforced cultural stereotypes that usually originated among white, male privilege groups. As Kenneth Woodrow and others have shown in research published in *Psychosomatic Medicine*, formulations such as 'men tolerate more pain than women' and 'Whites tolerate more pain than Orientals, while Blacks occupy an intermediate position' were commonplace, though they were refuted nearly as often as they were produced. It is striking the extent to which research in this vein still continues, with the primary quest being to discover a genetic explanation for variation in pain sensitivity, even though the analytical category in question is often not race at all, but ethnicity, which is not genetic but cultural. Even when such genetic research has been somewhat sensitive to cultural behaviour and identity, it nevertheless aimed to ascribe different pain signatures to different cultural groups in order to open up the possibility of ethnically tailored clinical pain treatment and management, thereby attempting to transform a cultural product into a fixed biomedical standard. Whether well intended or otherwise, these kinds of studies and opinions can be viewed as part of a politics of pain that has largely been constructed and controlled from within the medical and societal establishments of 'civilized' opinion. The history of such opinions about whose pain counts most and whose pain does not even register as pain at all has shown both a marked tendency to change over time as well as a lack of reflexivity concerning the assumptions and privileges that underlie such research. The onus on the pain validity of white, 'civilized' people has in many ways followed the changing discursive and material construction of civilization itself.

Urban nerves

The rise of the industrial city, and specifically of electrification, had a profound effect on the perceived nature of pain. Until the 1870s, throughout industrializing Europe, nervous illnesses had been bracketed as humoral imbalances, melancholy episodes, mania, and hysteria (Figure 7). These conditions, whether construed psychologically or, as in the case of hysteria, physiologically, were strongly gendered. They were especially female and, when occurring in men, were thought to be signs of effeminacy or sexual inversion. They tended to be treated outside of the strictly medical definitions of illness or disease. Insofar as these conditions were painful, it was generally understood that this 'pain' was not real, but 'in the mind', or else driven by a lack of emotional control under the influence of errant wombs and wanton libidinousness. These categories of mental and bodily disturbance went through changes in both nomenclature and gendering in the last quarter of the 19th century and through the first decades of the 20th, accelerated by the explosion of urban populations, mechanical innovations, and, most importantly, war.

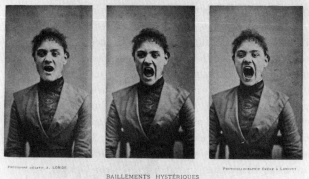

BAILLEMENTS HYSTÉRIQUES

7. Hysterical woman yawning, Nouvelle iconographie de la Salpêtrière (1890).

Modernity in civilization could itself be a threat to corporeal wellbeing. Victims of railway accidents who walked away without serious or lasting injuries nevertheless endured lasting manifestations of trauma that could not be definitively ascribed to the effects of physical lesions. 'Railway spine' was coined in the 1860s to define this new pathology, which was assumed to be an injury of the nervous system that science at that time could not see, but which must necessarily have existed. The notion of post-traumatic stress has slowly emerged from these roots, but with an important shift in emphasis. 'Railway spine' was either a mental aberration or a 'somatic' illness, with the latter view held especially by the leader in studies of the condition, John Eric Erichsen (1818–96). Irrespective of the fact that no physical or bodily pathology could be detected, he assumed that the body had been involved in physical forms of motion—the body incorporated into industrial forms of mechanical power—that had adversely affected it. Experts of nervous disorders were on the rise, looking for somatic explanations for emotional pain. There was no shortage of dissent, notably from Jean-Martin Charcot (1825–93)

Pain and civilization

in Paris, but new connections between body, nerves, and psychological trauma were being forged.

If (all too common) railway accidents provided a steady stream of patients, the condition of railway spine was still confined to a mere few. Of more general concern was the mass pathology of a growing bourgeoisie, with refined sensibilities, low tolerances for pain, and a susceptibility for being overwhelmed by the very environment that had produced, sustained, and captivated them. Cities were becoming electrified, lit at night. Stimulation of the senses and of the body was beyond an individual's control, with an onslaught of attraction and distraction coming twenty-four hours a day. The modern neurasthenic was born, being of a pathological nervous state, unable to cope with the pain induced by the complexities of urban and urbane existence. In the last decades of the 19th century, neurasthenia was typified by a host of ailments, from fatigue to headaches, high blood pressure, and low, brooding depressions. The strong gendering of hysterics as female gave way to a new order of nervous diseases that struck men and women alike. As industrial civilization, without a care for irony, drove its inhabitants into the slaughter of the First World War, nervous illness would increasingly be associated with combat trauma, and therefore men. The pains of civilization were, to those who suffered them, all too real and all too debilitating. But the history of civilization shows how pain was created, moved, invalidated, and validated, all the while shifting its ground and touching different groups. The high stakes of validation depended, to a large extent, on whether or not this pain or that could be entered into. The male hysteric of the 1880s was afforded little sympathy. By the 1920s, the same symptoms had a new pathology, a new set of treatments, and—for a while at least—the compassion of whole populations.

Chapter 5
Sympathy, compassion, empathy

In various ways we have already encountered sympathy and compassion as denoting a kind of suffering with, or of the taking of another's pain as one's own. 'Empathy' is a 20th-century coinage to describe similar phenomena. Sympathy and its correlates have played and continue to play an essential role in helping humans to determine who or what is in pain. The search in recent decades for proof of a biological empathy mechanism takes us into a neuroscientific adventure that looks for instruments in the human brain that would explain, according to the metaphors of electrical engineering and the hall of mirrors, how we can sense if someone else is in pain. But working out whose pain counts, which in turn determines whose pain is treated or ameliorated, and whose is ignored, depends upon the instrumentalization of sympathy or empathy. This is the root of a politics of pain.

Contexts of pain

One of the quirks of sympathy is that, as the capacity to recognize pain beyond our own body, we often recognize it where there can be no pain. We feel the pain that inheres in objects, in stories, and in noisy, dissonant sounds. The subject bears reflection because it helps to establish the social contingency of painful experience. Whatever the physiological and neurological constants of human experiences of others' pain, the causes of physiological and neurological stimulation are by no means fixed. The objects of sympathy change, sometimes over great expanses of time and place, but also in relatively short periods of our own experience. There is no definitive key to what suffering looks or sounds like.

Perhaps we have all experienced the onset of compassion fatigue. To some extent, this is represented by the news cycle, which zooms in on the human suffering caused by wars, natural disasters, and famine, but which loses our interest relatively quickly. Susan Sontag (1933–2004) highlighted the relative speed with which sympathy hardens into indifference, or even contempt, through the process of repeated exposure. We consume war through the lenses of cameras, to an extent that it becomes categorically indistinguishable from fictional accounts, designed to stir our emotions perhaps, but principally released to entertain us and loosen our wallets. What causes us pain one day may be a source of pleasure the next.

There is no more exemplary theatre of sympathetic fragility than the world of surgery. Scottish Enlightenment philosopher David Hume (1711–76) recognized in the 1730s that the capacity to sense pain somewhere or in someone else was dependent on recognizing the causes and effects of pain, not on being able to enter into a particular pain per se. He focused on surgery as a chief case in point. Anaesthetics were unknown, and the agonies of operations were a matter of common knowledge. Hume, imagining the surgical instruments, the bandages, the hot irons, and the anxiety of the patient and the operators, had his sympathies aroused, activated by pity and terror. Pain was implied, but not present. The causes were material. The effects were predictable and drawn from memory. In preparation for a major operation today, we would likely not be conscious of the material causes of pain, and nor would we experience any in an immediate sense. Put under general anaesthetic before arrival at the operating theatre, both patient and family are spared an examination of the medical instruments, and surgeons do not have to deal with the anguished faces and likely screams of their patients. We might, in the abstract, behold an 18th-century bone saw with indifference or even fascination. No terrors are here for us, let alone the well-spring of sympathy.

Pre-anaesthesia surgeons themselves were on constant guard with regard to being overwhelmed with sympathetic feelings. While the charge that surgeons became habitually callous to encounters with the pain of others are probably apocryphal, they did nevertheless have to retain a steady hand and an accomplished speed in order to minimize the trauma of their patients. Repetition was essential in forming a necessary habitual calm as part of 'professional' procedure. The discovery of chloroform and ether in the 1840s rapidly changed the surgeon's world. No longer did the material objects of the operating room have the capacity to arouse terror, simply because they could no longer be identified as causes of pain. Doubtless, the process of disassociation of surgical instruments and the sight of the opened and bloody body from the experience of pain was long and not always straightforward. But anaesthetic surgery provided the technological advance that allowed surgeons to practise with equanimity: steady hands, cool heads, calm nerves. For any students of surgery who found the prospect of practice unnerving, the famous Canadian physician William Osler (1849–1919) assured them in the 1880s that repetition would, for most, iron out the wrinkles of sympathetic pain. To betray fear or anxiety to a patient was to lose the patient's trust and confidence. 'Imperturbability' was the surgeon's watchword for it would save him (surgery was still an overwhelmingly male field in Osler's day) and his patient pain in the long run.

We can still see an awareness of the influence of the material causes of pain—that is, what they do to us emotionally before they have done anything physically—in contemporary medical practice. The World Health Organization (WHO) reported in October 2015 that pain at the time of vaccination is one of the most significant causes of anxiety for those who provide care to children. Concern that anxiety might actually hold caregivers back from having vaccinations carried out, the WHO put forward a series of recommendations to make sure the sympathies of onlookers were not over-stimulated. Vaccinators are instructed to remain calm, collaborate, be well informed, and use non-emotive language. Children are to be correctly positioned so that they don't have to see the needles, and the very young can be held by caregivers. It also recommends prior breastfeeding (where culturally accepted), and the ready availability of toys, videos, and the like as happy distractions. In short, the emotional atmosphere of the vaccinating station has to be transformed into a place that does not immediately indicate the primary purpose, namely vaccination. When the caregivers are less anxious, so the children vaccinated are themselves more liable to pick up on this mood and are therefore less likely to experience acute pain at the time of vaccination or immediately afterwards. Sympathy, then, is not only an emotional pain aroused in the observer by causes and effects of pain, but is also a potential transmitter of anxiety and fear that enhances pain. While in many instances sympathy with those in pain can help alleviate pain, in other instances it can make it worse.

Sympathy knowledge

The confusion about what sympathy is and how it works has confounded scholars for millennia. From Plato (d. 348/347 BCE) in classical antiquity to Max Scheler (1874–1928) at the beginning of the 20th century, and beyond, a working definition and functional explanation of the human capacity to feel someone else's pain has constantly shifted ground, as well as terminology. This capacity has been regarded as the basis of human civilization by such leading lights as the moral philosopher and political economist Adam Smith (1723–90) in the 18th century and Charles Darwin in the 19th. They did not exactly agree on what it was or how it worked, but they respectively marvelled—in their own ways—at its effects. There is broad agreement among evolutionary biologists that many species, including humans, have evolved an other-regarding instinct, but Darwin's observation in his *Descent of Man* (1871) that the later development of sympathy in humans depended upon 'public opinion' took the question into the realm of culture and politics. The problem is compounded when we consider how to map such a fuzzy concept onto other languages and other times. One English correlate for sympathy and compassion is 'pity', though its roots in Greek and Latin are distinct. In the Greek and Roman worlds, according to David Konstan in *Pity Transformed* (2001), pity was sufficiently polysemous to confound any reductive attempts to isolate a basic human trait, but it did nevertheless always have the capacity to indicate the pain or suffering of someone else, whether as *eleos* or *oiktos* in Greek, or as *misericordia* in Latin. But classical examples of pity—or its absence—should give us pause when trying to understand the objects of pity. Nothing is inherently or intrinsically pitiable. We might blench at ancient Greek treatment of, for example, prisoners of war, and label Greek generals as 'pitiless', but we would be anachronistic for so doing. Pity, like sympathy, overlays nature with context and politics. That is not to say, necessarily, that it is calculated. Political culture and political ethics are also, to a great degree, inscribed by nurture and habit. Throughout history, the withholding of mercy, pity, or compassion has been justified by the claim that a suffering *object*—be it a slave or an insect—was not worthy of clemency. Such discriminations are culturally bound, though we make them, and humans have always made them, as if they were natural.

Sympathy's importance as a social phenomenon reached its apogee in the 18th century, with various eminent philosophers contributing arguments about the centrality of perceptions of suffering to the functioning of civilization. Adam Smith, David Hume, and Edmund Burke (1729–97), the philosopher and statesman, foregrounded sympathy in their respective accounts of the ways in which society hung together and fell apart. For Smith, whose work was probably the most influential, sympathy was a social bond that distinguished civilized societies from more 'primitive' cultures. The capacity for individuals mutually to enter into one another's emotional experiences was the essential foundation for both moral behaviour and social action. Understanding someone else's feelings was considered to be an essential guide to good conduct, since acting out of sympathy for others would likely lead others to act out of sympathy in return. To offer succour for emotional pain was a way of ensuring that such succour would be returned to you in a time of need. Sympathy, for the likes of Smith, facilitated the Golden Rule, at the centre of which was the self.

As the late 18th century became increasingly preoccupied with questions of liberty and with Utilitarian equations of pleasure and pain, so the capacity to understand who was suffering and why came to be at the very centre of ethics and political economy. By the mid-19th century, utilitarian philosopher John Stuart Mill (1806–73), in his *On Liberty* (1859), could formulate this 'harm principle' as follows: 'The only purpose for which power can be rightfully exercised over any member of a civilized community, against his will, is to prevent harm to others'. The assumption here (glossing over the reference to 'civilized communities', about which I refer the reader to Chapter 4), is that 'harm'—hurt, pain, suffering, *injury* in the broadest sense—is both identifiable and can be legislated against. It also provides a code of personal conduct that assumes that an individual will recognize when her actions are causing harm to others and therefore change her behaviour. A general appreciation of *hurt* became the guiding principle for moral conduct.

In the same year that Mill published *On Liberty*, Charles Darwin published *On the Origin of Species* (1859). Darwin would go on to challenge the construction of sympathy he found in Smith and Mill, denying that acts of sympathy to alleviate suffering had to be intentional in order to be moral. For Darwin, the most successful societies had succeeded precisely because their sympathetic instincts (and therefore their morals) were built in. Primitive societies that were built on the alleviation of the suffering of neighbours had come into existence through evolution. They were moral by nature, with their progress toward civilization reinforced by culture. Darwin and some of his followers hoped that the apex of civilization would herald the end of the struggle for existence: a human triumph over a state of nature in which only the fittest survived and the existence of the majority was defined by pain and suffering. That triumph, were it to come, was to be built on an ever increasing capacity for and refinement of sympathy. With the ticking over of the 19th century into the 20th, so the focus shifted from sympathy to empathy, and the quest to understand the nature of the human capacity to enter into the sufferings of others.

While Darwin's vision has been somewhat lost, the notion of a built-in sense of the sufferings of others has inspired continuous research ever since. Work in this area is connected to more general studies of theory of mind, which aim to understand human and animal capacities for recognizing their own minds and the minds of others, and what leads to failure of such capacities in some individuals. Though the mind is immaterial, some cognitive scientists have tried to locate the specific brain 'mechanisms' involved in theory of mind by employing neuroimaging devices. Functional MRI scanners are able to detect changes in the blood oxygen level in parts of the brain that correspond to neural activity. The results are processed in order to form maps that show which parts of the brain particularly 'light up' when performing a task, thinking about such a task, viewing images, hearing sounds, etc. Empathy research, which more specifically explores by what means the brain enters into the pains and emotions of others, has turned to such neuroimaging techniques.

The 'wiring' of empathy

What is the functional connection or overlap between the neural pathways involved in sensing and combating physical pain and those that sense and experience the pain of others? This pain/ empathy concordance has been tested on the basis of a hypothesis that witnessing pain had similar physiological effects to experiencing pain directly. To a certain extent, the research bore out the hypothesis, showing that the endogenous opioid systems in the brain—that is, the brain's natural painkillers—were engaged by seeing images of others in pain, just as they would be in the event of an injury directly to the body. Neuroscientists' search for the 'mechanisms' of both pain and empathy are complemented by perspectives from the social sciences as the two fields become increasingly intertwined. *Longue durée* and cross-cultural perspectives show that neither the experience of pain nor of empathy is a constant among humans. When and how they appear are contingent on contextual understandings and definitions, even if they can be isolated as physiological constants in many mammals, including humans.

If a test subject looks at images of people suffering in order to gauge his response, the assumption is that the subject already understands what suffering looks like. There is good reason to assume this within certain limits, based on cultural and temporal affinity, but outside these limits conscious empathy is not guaranteed. A failure of empathic brain activity when confronted with an image of suffering might indicate theory of mind impairment consistent with autism spectrum disorders. But a person's inability to recognize that suffering is taking place, or that such suffering is likely to happen to us, might also be an indicator that the appropriate cultural scripts are missing. The latter was essential to Aristotle's definition of pity, which was a 'kind of pain' arising only when a species of suffering in someone else was recognized as a potential threat to the self. A number of studies have shown that empathy is dependent on our ability to call forth emotions that we have experienced first-hand, or on our capacity to imagine being in the other's shoes. Since the situational arousal of emotion depends on temporal and cultural contexts as well as on our physiology, our capacity to empathize is limited to that which we can readily translate into an experience of our own. This might be highly successful, or an empathic experience might be significantly different to the pain/emotion observed.

Neuroscientific research has looked for the 'hard-wiring' of empathy in the brain. The discovery of 'mirror neurons' has generated a great deal of controversy among the neuroscientific community. These neurons are supposed to be activated by observing an action of another individual, just as they would be if the witness were performing the same action herself. In other words, mirror neurons collapse the distance between you and me. When your actions fire my mirror neurons, it is as if I am carrying out those actions myself. Mirror neurons have therefore become key to understanding how theory of mind capacities work. A degree of scepticism still surrounds this research, in part focusing on whether findings on brain activity related to hand actions in monkeys can be extrapolated to emotional brain activity in humans. Assuming such internal 'mirrors' do exist and function as described—and indeed there is a growing body of work in support of the theory—there are still limits to its implications. What happens when we encounter emotional expressions that are alien to us? What happens when the mirror that society holds up to us does not compute with our own idea of ourselves? We can and do carry out interpretive or translation work, but within limits. Although there are well-documented constants with respect to what fear or disgust look or feel like, there is also persuasive research that demonstrates a lack of universal elicitors of these emotions. Objects and expressions derive their meanings through experience and through cultural ascriptions that are taught, learned, and mutually reinforced through communities of common feeling and understanding. To recognize what is painful—for mirror neurons to function—is to be involved in, or to try to enter, an intricate web of cultural signs and symbols.

Empathy in context

Various historical narratives have emphasized this phenomenon, where new ideas about suffering have not yet reached a commonly accepted level of understanding and recognition. The 18th-century wave of activism that saw the rise of anti-slavery movements and the beginnings of animal welfarism, to cite just two examples, had to reckon with the intransigence of most people to the emergence of new ethical concerns. Both movements had to do something to the status and meaning of their subjects of concern (slaves and animals), not the least of which was to make them *subjects* instead of mere instrumental objects. The beating of an animal may have indicated a kind of callousness on the part of the human doing the beating, but it is unlikely that a witness to such an event would have felt 'empathy' with the animal as we might, since no concept of suffering on its part would have registered. Similarly with slaves, essential to the success of the movement to abolish the slave trade was the elevation of slaves to the category of humanity. Viewing them as something categorically *other* resulted in no compunction about their mistreatment.

To take this a stage further, it is worth remembering that the campaign to abolish slavery and the early campaigns to protect animals from cruelty took place in a context of vast social inequality, wage slavery, and urban poverty. If we could visit the slums of major cities in the first decade of the 19th century we, no doubt, would empathize profoundly with the suffering of the urban poor at the heart of the so-called 'civilized world'. That contemporary reformers were not so activated has puzzled historians, who have struggled to explain why the suffering of class others did not resonate with reformers to the same extent as the sufferings of race others and species others. One persuasive theory, first put forward by historian Thomas Haskell in 1985, postulates that one can only see, or acknowledge, suffering when a moral compunction to help is coupled with feasible and relatively easy strategies of assistance. A popular view held that whereas slaves and animals had had their lot forced upon them, the indolent masses (as the better-off saw them) only had themselves to blame for their hardship. For many, the problem of inequality was neither a moral quandary nor an easy fix, and the poor therefore remained outside the boundaries of emotional concern. In other words, to suffer with someone—to be sympathetic or compassionate—implies that there is the possibility, at the individual or societal level, of offering succour, as well as a sense of moral duty to follow through. As circumstances change, so possibilities change too. The neural 'mechanisms' of empathy may be built in, but what activates them is not. When looking for empathy failure, therefore, we might do well to look at the cultural *mise en scène*.

The neurochemical advances in our understanding of both pain and empathy have profound implications for our experience of pain in the world. If pain and empathy are functionally related—that is, being in pain and witnessing another in pain—then taking pain medication designed to eliminate physical pain might also eliminate the emotional pain caused by witnessing suffering. In fact, the functional correspondence offers scientific weight to the slow collapse of the distinction between the physical and the emotional. While the research on empathic pain is at the cutting edge of neuroscience, neuropsychologists and human geneticists have argued for some time that individual emotional suffering, caused perhaps by social exclusion, bereavement, or a 'broken heart', is neurologically no different to (or at least has much in common with) pains caused by injury. Geneticists have isolated genetic variants that correspond to a higher likelihood to suffer 'social pain', in accordance with fMRI work that demonstrates the presence of pain responses in situations designed to elicit negative emotional reactions. Moreover, a number of researchers have confirmed in a wide variety of studies that regular pain killers (acetaminophen, for example) combat this emotional pain. For those genetically predisposed to suffer, a regular regimen of acetaminophen at low doses has been shown to improve social adjustment and reduce feelings of social or emotional pain. Correspondingly, a regular dose of acetaminophen has been shown to reduce empathetic responses to images of suffering, with implications both potentially negative and positive.

The ability to turn off or at least limit the 'volume' of empathy would doubtless be useful to those who are faced with having to work efficiently in traumatic situations (such as doctors and journalists in war zones), while the numbing of emotional pain among those most susceptible to it may also limit their capacity to feel the pain of others. We may also have to change our vocabulary when considering individuals who do not have a high capacity to empathize with others. Instead of thinking in terms of a mechanical empathy failure, we might think in terms of 'empathy analgesia'. Recent research has indeed shown that the administration of opioid antagonists—that is, drugs to prevent the body's natural painkillers from working properly—increases the empathic capacities of test subjects. A heightened sensitivity to painful injury therefore probably equates to a more acute sense of the sufferings of others.

Chapter 6
Pain as pleasure

There have been numerous attempts in modernity to make the claim that all pain is evil. Utilitarians in the 19th century did so, and neo-utilitarians from the late 20th century to the present, such as Richard Ryder (b. 1940), continue to do so. In Ryder's case, involvement in animal research prompted an extreme aversion to any kind of suffering, particularly in animals. Pain has been conceptualized as always a malign experience that should be reduced or eliminated. Yet, as we have seen, many cultures and traditions have the pursuit or acceptance of pain as a central part of virtuous existence, from asceticism to the ultimate extreme of martyrdom. And from a functional point of view too, there are compelling reasons why pain is essential and helpful. Without pain, as anyone with congenital analgesia will attest, we are at enormous risk. Pain holds us in check when there is something wrong, causing us to protect injured parts. Limping on a twisted ankle isn't a sign of injury but a sign of recovery. If we did not feel the pain we would make the ankle bear our load and the ankle, without being guarded, would soon deteriorate. Pain is necessary, from an evolutionary and individual standpoint, for it aids survival. This is not so much the story of our acute reflexes to painful stimuli as it is the story of our ongoing protective reflexes to enduring states of pain after injury. In this most fundamental sense, the potential for dysfunction notwithstanding, pain is an unmitigated good. All this notwithstanding, when pain has been sought explicitly as pleasure, it has been viewed by some as immoral, perverse, or indicative of mental illness.

Looking at pain

What could it mean to experience pain as pleasure? Is this dysfunction? A line-up of notorious sado-masochists might inspire us to answer in the affirmative, but this is not the whole story. Nor does it boil down to a simple thrill of *Schadenfreude* as the clown takes a spill on a banana skin. Even if the very idea of experiencing pain—one's own or someone else's—as pleasure is disconcerting, philosophers since Plato have not only acknowledged its existence, but also attested to its being a fundamental quality of humanity. The Ghazal poets of South Asia, whose couplets since the 12th century have captured the unbearable pain of unattainable love while at the same time acknowledging love's splendour, knew this. Long-distance runners have also testified anecdotally about the 'runner's high', a feeling of euphoria achieved through the severe pain of having run marathon distances and farther. Neuroimaging research has begun to confirm what those runners know: euphoria is enhanced through running by changing the way that opioids are processed in the brain. But what about deriving pleasure from looking at pain?

In 2003 Susan Sontag wondered at some length in *Regarding the Pain of Others* at the power of the photograph of suffering to hold our attention. Why do we take and consume pictures of pain? The answer is complex, but a fundamental part of it is that we feel compelled to look. Other people's pain is ugly, disgusting, repulsive. In the abstract, we turn away. But then we turn back. Pain is profane and, like most taboos, attractive *because* it isn't supposed to be. Just as we slow to a crawl to look at a car accident—Sontag dismisses a pure curiosity in favour of a genuine desire 'to see something gruesome'—we also pause to observe a person being loaded into the back of an ambulance on a gurney.

If we are filled with an abstract concern, we are equally filled with an abstract desire to see injury, distress, even death. Disgust at the aesthetics of pain, and the fear aroused by putting oneself in the place of the sufferer, ought to drive us from the scene. But disgust and fear, insofar as they are visually inspired, demand to be looked at. How else are we to know what disgusts or frightens us? Thus we are rooted, enquiring, but also enjoying the pain of others.

This paradox has been widely observed. Sigmund Freud, the pioneering psychoanalyst, made a career out of it. Plato, in the *Republic* (*c*.380 BCE), has Socrates recount the story of Leontius giving in to the desire to look at dead bodies. Edmund Burke, in *A Philosophical Enquiry into the Origin of Our Ideas of the Sublime and Beautiful* (1757), elides pain and fear when the fear is one's own. But when the fear, or terror, is somebody else's, it is experienced as a mixture, according to Jan Mieszkowski's 2012 reading of Burke, of 'pity and pleasure, of pain and delight'. We approach the experience of the sublime. The reasoning is clear enough: when we are put to an active purpose, we are imbued with delight or pleasure. If the recognition of another's pain were only ever painful to the observer, the observer would do all he could to avoid the sights of suffering. But we seek out such sights for the curious admixture of delight and distress. If we are thus compelled to relieve the pain of the suffering we see, it is perhaps first and foremost to relieve it in ourselves, and this is only a heightening of the pleasure that was activated in us when we first beheld the pain. Sympathy, humanity, compassion—call it what you will—has throughout history been thought of as a self-serving activity in equal measure to being an other-serving activity.

Toward the end of the 19th century, some philosophers (or proto social scientists) sought to reverse this 'ego-altruism', as Herbert Spencer (1820–1903) called it. He highlighted the tendency of people to 'luxuriate' in pity, an indulgence in the suffering of others akin to the trite effect of big eyes on a baby seal. Pity is a curious pain/pleasure emotion. It depends on the pain of others (self-pity is usually derided as self-indulgent wallowing), but is also a necessary human quality. A person without pity is reviled as a monster. How are we to know who these monsters are, or if we ourselves are monsters, unless there is pain? In this respect, pain seems to have been a remarkably persistent social building block.

Divine pain

If this seems far-fetched, what are we to make of figures who seem genuinely to have relished being in or witnessing pain? The Carmelite nun and Spanish mystic, Teresa of Ávila (1515–82; canonized, 1622) experienced such ecstatic pain that one might wonder if the pain she described was anything akin to pain as we know it. She is typically depicted in the presence of the Trinity as a dove, being pierced in the heart with an arrow or spear, delivered by a fiery angel. Artistic renderings of Teresa's facial expression tend towards swooning pleasure, almost orgasmic ecstasy. Many artists followed the lead of Bernini's (1598–1680) *Ecstasy of Saint Teresa* (1647–52), which showed Teresa in ecstasy in the moment immediately prior to being penetrated with a spear. Her own description of this moment was the direct inspiration for the way she is generally depicted in painting and sculpture. As the angel withdrew his spear he drew out her entrails, leaving her 'completely afire with a great love for God. The pain was so sharp that it made me utter several moans; and so excessive was the sweetness caused me by the intense pain that one can never wish to lose it'. Teresa's pain was not merely of the body, but, as she experienced it, of the soul. As Maria Berbara, a scholar of Teresa, points out, she was as annoyed and troubled by quotidian physical pain as the next person. But this deeply symbolic, religious experience of pain, with its accompanying vision, was, in its excruciating nature, a coming together with God.

Teresa was far from alone in connecting an acutely painful experience with a moment of ecstasy, and we should be cautious in inferring something crudely erotic. Clemente Susini's (1754–1814)

Venere dei Medici (1780–2) is a wax anatomical model of a young woman in the last moment of life. The lithe naked frame of this woman is shown arched, not in pain, but in ecstasy. This position is rendered uncanny by the fact that her skin from pubis to thorax has been cut away, revealing her internal organs, which are themselves removable in layers. It is at once erotic and sensual, morbid and gory. The Poggi Palace in Bologna, which preserves a historical replica, itself describes this 'alienating effect' as the problem of our gaze, since the rationale behind the model focuses on the 'sensitivity' of the human who gives herself up to death. If there is pain represented here—and we might wonder how it could be otherwise—then it is indistinguishable from an ecstatic serenity.

In his 2013 work, *Pain, Pleasure and Perversity*, John Yamamoto-Wilson makes the point that, in a world in which pain and suffering were everywhere, and where suffering was constructed as a virtue—a divine bestowal of pain as a reward for sin, and as a down payment for time in purgatory—the concept of masochism hardly needed to be explicitly defined. Everybody was a masochist, in a sense, making use of their pain and translating it into a sort of divinely instilled joy. The Reformation changed this by denying the purificatory action of pain with respect to sin. To enjoy pain even though it was of no use emerged as a perversion only once the theological purpose of pain had been demolished. The fact that Eros had probably already been aroused through the disciplinary practices of a number of Catholic Orders was a priori evidence, in the Protestant world, of a sexual vice implicit in the seeking out of pain.

Pain and sex

The Protestant world would have ample opportunity to disapprove of this sexual vice in the realms of English schooling. The centrality of 'discipline'—the rod and the birch—to pedagogy had unlooked for consequences, both among teachers and pupils.

The association of pain and sexual pleasure in this context was first observed in English in 1676, in Thomas Shadwell's (1642–92) play, *The Virtuoso*. Amidst a complex entanglement of love interests, sexual misdemeanour, and bawdy smut, the character Snarl has a penchant for the rod, carried over from school life. Spanking and caning garnered the colloquial assignation, 'the English vice' in 19th-century France. After Shadwell, there were frequent cultural references to sexual pleasure derived from pain, even if the practice had not been formally named. In *Fanny Hill* (1748/9), one Mr Barville can only enjoy sex while being whipped or whipping alike, a phenomenon captured photographically by the pioneering sexologist Richard von Krafft Ebing (1840–1902) towards the end of the 19th century (Figure 8). Here was a man, according to Fanny, 'condemned to have his pleasure lashed into him, as boys have their learning'. Close in date to Fanny's adventures was William Hogarth's (1697–1764) *Harlot's Progress* (1732), the third stage of which clearly depicts a birch hanging on the wall behind Moll Hackabout's bed-as-place-of-work, along with a witch's hat. Her feline familiar, striking a pose of readiness for sexual reception, completes a scene that associates the whore with the demonic. What is striking about these kinds of examples is not only the readily understood and possibly even unsurprising appearances of pain as sexual pleasure, but also the unbreakable association of what would have been deemed a perverse pathology with the most licentious, immoral, and degrading of scenes. Nevertheless, both *Fanny Hill* and *The Harlot's Progress* did a brisk trade.

Various scholars have tried to theorize why pain might be pleasurable, even ecstatic, since the early 17th century. Johann Heinrich Meibom (1590–1655) offered a treatise on the subject in Latin in 1629, in the time-honoured fashion of hiding explicit subjects in the language of the learned: *De flagrorum usu in re veneria*. Appearing over a century before the birth of the Marquis de Sade, it is testimony to the much older roots of what would come to be commonly known as 'sadism'. The 1761 English

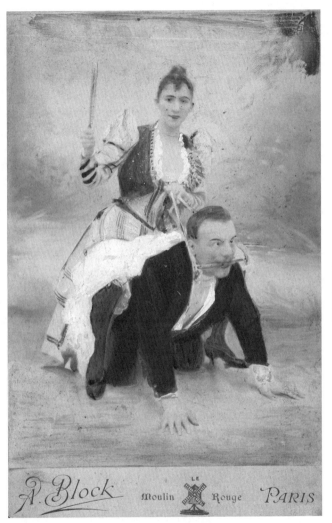

8. Richard von Kraft-Ebing, *Man on all fours in red jacket with clothed woman riding him and holding a whip* (c.1896).

translation of the work, *A Treatise of the Use of Flogging in Venereal Affairs*, made plain the extraordinary accounts of 'persons who are stimulated to venery by strokes of the rod, and worked into a flame of lust by blows; and that the part, which distinguishes us to be men, should be raised by the charm of invigorating lashes'. Meibom traces such practices to as far back as Picus, mythical first king of Latium, and argues that such things become customary once introduced, as if second nature. But adding a lengthy physiological explanation, he opines that the kidneys are essential to the production of 'seed', and that lecherous types and those 'exhausted by too frequent a repetition' seek a 'remedy by flogging'. In being beaten, heat is excited in the

> seminal matter, and that more particularly from the pain of the
> flogged parts, which is the reason that the blood and spirits are
> attracted in a greater quantity, till the heat is communicated
> to the organs of generation, and the perverse and frenzical
> appetite is satisfied.

That is not an explanation that has endured, though the notion of custom is important. It is probable that anticipation of sexual pleasure through painful processes makes for a favourable context of fulfilment. The long history of ecstasy through pain is further evidence of the lack of a direct relationship between injury and the unpleasantness we usually call pain. Sado-masochistic practices highlight the extent to which the meaningfulness of pain—the affective constructions of significance that take place in the brain and in the context of the world at a given moment—is endlessly variable. Injury, when coupled with fear, anxiety, and a feeling of being out of control, can make pain unbearable. Yet injury, when coupled with trust, pleasure, and the anticipation of sexual ecstasy, can make pain a truly welcome bedfellow.

There is evidence of complicit receipt of pain that goes as far back as the *Kama Sutra*, which is at least 1,800 years old. Chapter five of the 1883 English translation begins: 'All the places that can be kissed are also the places that can be bitten, except the upper lip, the interior of the mouth, and the eyes'. There are numerous historical, erotic cultures of pain as pleasure, Japanese Kinbaku/ Shibari rope bondage being one example that continues to be practised today. Shibari is an art form and erotic practice adapted from Samurai Hojōjutsu techniques of prisoner restraint. It involves a dynamic relationship of Nawashi (rope master) and consenting model or partner, who is bound. The ropes are tied in such a way as to activate erogenous zones. The situation is defined by a complex relationship of power, pain, pleasure, and Eros.

Masochism receives its archetypical expression in Leopold von Sacher-Masoch's (1836–95) 1870 work *Venus im Pelz* (*Venus in Furs*), in which we follow the self-abandonment of Severin, who willingly becomes the slave of Wanda. The imagery of *Venus im Pelz* is profoundly drawn from the Catholic canon of martyrology and of historical practices of flagellation and discipline. Severin's fantasies are forged in accounts of the joyous pains of martyrs, and Wanda warns him to be careful lest he become the martyr of a woman. At one point, Wanda tells him how wonderful he would look if he were being beaten to death in agony, with his 'eye of a martyr'. The chief instrument of Wanda's domination is the whip, as Severin suffers bound to a post. Yet such allusions to a saintly or devotional path are constantly subverted by a context devoid of religiosity. Wanda herself is Venus, a pagan goddess, and her acquiescence to Severin's scheme of slavery is based on a classical cosmology of beauty and bondage. Severin himself is, by his own admission, in need of a 'cure'. His need to be enslaved is a pathology curable only through the enslavement (and betrayal) itself. The cornerstone of masochistic culture is built on such paradoxes. Hate, jealousy, and pain are conceived and experienced as love, joy, and pleasure, and while Severin repeatedly exclaims the heartlessness and evil of his tormentor, in so doing he is only drawn further into her power. Here pain becomes the instrument not only of sexual arousal and fulfilment, but also a bond of attachment. Unable to co-exist as equals—this is the explicitly stated structural dynamic of gender relations—the choice is only to conquer or be conquered. The whip, the heel, the forced confinement, the yoking to a plough—all these methods of inflicting pain and of experiencing pain serve to affirm and re-affirm the bond that Severin willingly signs between slave and master. While his torment drives him almost to suicide, it is only through pain that Severin can make his bond—his love—with Wanda tangible. His pain and suffering is terrible, terrifying, ecstatic, and proof of love.

Sexology

Pain

The allusions to animalistic behaviour formed the basis of some attempts to explain why pain and pleasure, or more particularly pain and sex, went hand in hand. The reputed pioneering sexologist, Havelock Ellis (1859–1939), alluded in 1903 to the mammalian animality of humanity to account for the 'intimate and inevitable association...of combat...with the process of courtship' in order to account for love's 'close connection with pain'. Evolutionary hangovers were, in his opinion, nevertheless corrupted by civilization, to the point that female pleasure became neglected and the expression of male power (and therefore cruelty) flowed without check. Somewhat incongruously, women were thought to derive pleasure through submission, also as a 'normal' result of development from animal rituals of courtship. 'Normal' sexual relations were only the preface to Ellis's greater interests in the 'region of the morbid', which had also activated and animated the growing band of professional psychologists and psychiatrists. One such, the German Albert von Schrenck-Notzing (1862–1929), tried to re-classify sado-masochism according to its barest terms, namely, sexual excitement in and through pain. As with most intellectual neologisms of the late 19th century, Schrenck-Notzing plumped for a Greek compound: algolagnia.

It didn't catch on, but the reality of sexual pleasure derived through pain—either in its infliction or in its reception—was firmly established. Moreover, for experts like Ellis, it was either within the bounds of normalcy or at least close by, observable in nature and explainable in humans. As for flagellation, or 'discipline', the overlap of nervous fibres between the buttocks and the genitals went some way to explaining the phenomenon of this specific pain-pleasure phenomenon. And for sado-masochists, Ellis above all established that the specific pleasure principle was connected to pain explicitly, rather than cruelty or domination. The reason? Ellis summed it up thus: 'Pain acts as a sexual stimulant because it is the most powerful of all methods for arousing emotion'. Specifically, Ellis recognized that in pain we are also in anger or fear, and that these emotions suffuse our pain with meaning. Connecting such feelings again to evolutionary models of development, he postulated that they were not alien to sexual life, but indeed intimately bound up with sexual selection. Latent in the 'normal', they were more closely associated with sexual action in those who crossed into 'abnormal' realms. In the specific context of coitus, male anger and female fear were themselves articles of pleasure, aroused specifically through pain. In the neuropathic, pain became an 'indispensable stimulant to the sexual system'.

Many cultures today have dispensed with the early 20th century's distinctions of 'normal' and 'abnormal', and live in a world in which the sexual pleasure of pain has become a commonplace article of popular culture. Even if it is concluded that actual first-hand participation in sado-masochistic acts is a minority pursuit, the runaway success of *Fifty Shades of Grey* (2011) by E.L. James (b. 1963) has shown without a doubt that there exists an overwhelming public interest in the consumption of painful pleasure. We might formulate that as an elaborate contrivance to derive pleasure from witnessing pain. Regardless of what we call it, the existence of painful pleasure and its apparent lack of connection to medical discourses of the function and meaning, or the problem, of pain, should give us pause. If nothing else, it shows us the central importance of emotions, or affective states, in determining the meaning of pain and the way in which it is experienced. What happens when that knowledge is re-applied to medical attempts both to understand and to eliminate pain?

Chapter 7
Pain in modern medicine and science

Nociception

Contemporary medicine strives for diagnosis, definition, certainty. While the history of pain suggests that we should avoid linguistic reductions and Anglophone chauvinism, the IASP thought it essential to define the terms of its study. The definition is being tested by pain scholars—sociologists, phenomenologists, and bioethicists—who challenge the continued dualism that pervades contemporary medical practice, and who demonstrate that the focus on injury (or the potential for it) is causing medicine to overlook millions of people in pain who feel unable to turn to medicine for help. Even if emotional pain is regarded as legitimate or authentic, to continue with distinct notions of emotional pain and physical pain perpetuates the dualism that denies the interrelation and interdependence of the two. We are not, so the argument goes, dealing with two distinct concepts in physical and emotional pain, but one.

That it remains so apparently easy to divide them, as psychologist Robert Kugelmann pointed out in 2000, is a result of 'sedimented cultural categories...for carving up the person into psyche and soma'. Patrick Wall frequently lamented the paucity of knowledge among doctors of the nature/culture of pain. Medical students' study of pain is often limited to a focus on the diagnosis and treatment of injury and disease. Judy Foreman, in *A Nation in Pain* (2014), found that neither pain biology nor 'modern principles of pain relief and palliative care' are taught to medical students across 80 per cent of the world. A roughly Cartesian statement that describes an injurious stimulus, a 'nociceptive' nerve-ending, a signal of *pain*, and the receipt of this signal in the brain, which then determines a series of reactions to the pain signal, is still pervasive among the medical community. I parenthesize the word 'nociceptive', and emphasize the word *pain* because both are erroneous, if useful nonetheless, rhetorical commonplaces.

First of all, the nerve endings in the skin respond not to pain, but to many levels of touch and temperature or chemical stimulation, including that which is injurious. The signals sent through the central nervous system to the brain in the case of damage are not 'pain' signals, but injury signals. 'Nociception', from the Latin *nocere*, might be correct if taken to mean 'detection of harm', but it is usually taken to mean 'detection of hurt', and the nerves that detect harm are called either 'nociceptors' or 'pain receptors'. Yet there is nothing in nociception that necessitates the experience of pain.

What is happening on a physiological level in the event of injury is the body's attempt to restore homeostasis. A disruption to normal functions, or neurological activity, of temperature, of chemical 'balance', leads to automatic responses to restore the body's internal conditions to 'normal'. All these physiological reactions potentially play a part in the experience of pain, but in and of themselves they are not pain. They may create the bodily conditions that are interpreted in the brain as pain, but they do not determine the magnitude, duration, or unpleasantness of it.

The focus here on acute injury gives us a clue as to why 'nociception' has proven so persuasive and enduring as *the* description of pain. There is something so inescapably logical and obvious about the notion of a pain pathway. The image of pulling the foot from the fire is, completely unthinkingly, animated in our minds by the addition of a vocal utterance: 'Ow!' Anyone who has ever cut himself on a kitchen knife, or touched a hot pan, or stubbed a toe, knows the natural association of injurious stimulus and pain. But we must remember that in this kind of situation we are immediately and certainly conscious of what we have done, attending to context and circumstance. We imbue the damage, especially the sight of the damage, with all of its potential harmful implications. Pain experience is formed within all of this immediately available knowledge and awareness. Change the scene: many people who suffer gun-shot wounds claim to have been unaware, at the moment of being shot, of any pain. Pain may only arrive once the victim realizes what has happened to her. Likewise, soldiers with severe battle trauma, car-crash victims, and all manner of other individuals with major tissue damage claim to have felt no pain at the time of their injuries, or even for some time afterwards. Add these mysterious absences of pain to all those cases of recurring pain, chronic pain, and emotional pain, where there is no obvious nociception to explain why it hurts, and we realize that this historically persuasive and oft-repeated interpretation of how pain functions is inadequate.

Gate control theory

Modern medicine persisted with a dualistic approach to pain for a remarkably long time, and it is important to distinguish medical approaches to, and understandings of, pain from medical advances in anaesthesia. The 'modern' approach to pain is usually associated with the medical adoption of chloroform and ether from the 1840s. Indeed, this was a remarkable innovation, both in terms of patient experiences of surgery and for the development of surgical practices deemed too extreme for the conscious patient. But for all the procedural advantages of anaesthesia, it only reinforced traditional separations of bodily sensation and mental disturbance, and it did very little if anything for those suffering from chronic pain. Anaesthetic temporarily shut off sensation, but did not immediately further the understanding of what pain was or how it worked.

In the 1960s, Melzack and Wall became increasingly alarmed by what they perceived as the profound ignorance of pain, pain states, and pain management within the medical establishment and among those practitioners who encountered pain on a daily basis. They recognized that the pain theories that guided the action of medical practitioners did not accurately describe what they themselves witnessed in their treatment of people in pain. The simple notions of a pain pathway and of a direct correlation between magnitude of injury and magnitude of pain were both manifestly false. A new theory was required that would explain the variability of pain experience, opening the door to the role of the brain and of affect in regulating (or failing to regulate) the experience of pain.

They came up with the 'gate control theory' of pain in 1965, which in turn revolutionized pain research (Figure 9). The theory was simple enough, describing a 'gate' in the spinal cord through which signals from the periphery have to pass in order to tell the brain about injury. Three different types of nerve fibre that respond to different magnitudes of stimulation are received in the gate control. The combined 'message' of those signals partly determines what gets transmitted to the brain and what signals are inhibited. The gate control is also the recipient of descending signals from the brain that regulate experience. This theory combined elements of older theories that had designated specific functions for specific nerves, and the patterning of nervous signals in the overall delivery of 'pain' signals. Importantly, the theory's postulation of different types of nervous involvement in pain processing did away with the search for a specific 'nociceptor' or nerve with the specific function of sending pain messages. Rather, the new theory described how nerves with different firing thresholds were mutually involved in the regulation of which

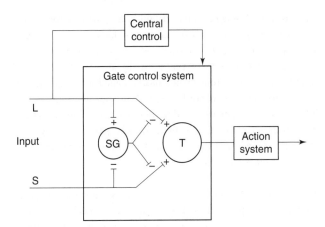

9. Gate control mechanism (1965).

signals were transmitted from the spinal cord to the brain.
Melzack and Wall went a step further in describing how the
magnitude and type of nervous stimulation, the brain's evaluative
assessment of the context, and the emotional state of the subject
determined when and which 'pain' signals were allowed through
the gate control.

There were additional nuances that helped plug the gaps in
prevailing theories of pain. Signalling from within the spinal cord
itself, even after the signalling from the periphery had ceased,
accounted for otherwise inexplicable cases of enduring pain after
injury, and the tendency to mislocate where pain was occurring in
the body. Moreover, it was theorized that the signals ascending
and descending into the gate control were potentially self-
sustaining, involved in a reactionary relationship that could
sustain painful experience long after an injury. The multiple
involvement of different types of nerve could also explain types
of sensory dysfunction. Sensitization using capsaicin, for example,
has demonstrated that thresholds of sensitivity to heat and cold
can be manipulated, with 'burning' occurring at innocuous

temperatures. Using the same irritant in larger doses over time has the opposite effect of overloading and 'knocking out' these 'nociceptors', having an anaesthetic effect. Certain nerves (C fibres and A delta fibres) that normally carry injury signals can be fired by mere touch when in a damaged state. An ongoing excitability can cause central sensitization, meaning that inhibition in the gate control does not take place. Under these conditions, a person might suffer allodynia (pain caused by stimuli that ought not to be noxious) and hyperalgesia (an abnormal sensitivity to pain).

The gate control theory unlocked many mysteries, affording the possibility to explore the body's own inhibitory mechanisms in regulating pain. Not the least of these was the role of affect or emotion in determining the unpleasantness of pain. There were problems with the gate control theory, however. It furthered our understanding of the variability of pain states after acute injury, but it did not adequately describe chronic pain, or pain when there was no lesion (and never had been). Moreover, as research into pain 'mechanisms'—and the gate control was certainly a mechanism—proliferated, the language of the pain pathway endured. In other words, the messages being regulated in the gate control have been understood as 'pain' messages, sent from the periphery or sustained in the spinal cord.

Sensational pathways

The concept of a pain pathway is remarkably tenacious. Even among those who know that pain is not reducible to injury, or, to put it another way, that pain cannot be explained solely by nervous signals sent from the periphery to the brain, the idea of a pathway lingers. The human being still gets rhetorically chopped up into separate body and mind entities, with corresponding strands of research that are respectively limited to the nervous system and the mind. The confusion is easy enough to explain, in part because it is our intuitive understanding of what is happening to us when we experience an acute injury, which is the easiest kind of pain to imagine.

When I was five, I was left alone in my grandmother's parlour, watching an open fire. I put the iron poker in the hottest part of the fire and left it there until it started to glow red. An inescapable curiosity compelled me to find out what this 'red' was like, so I pinched the poker end between finger and thumb. It produced, in a short time, two white blisters. What was happening at the moment of grasping and releasing the poker would classically be described as follows. By way of reflex I immediately let go of the poker and turned my attention to my fingers, looking at them intently. A cascade of signals was immediately sent from the skin of the fingertips to the central nervous system. In very short order, as a response to the detection of injury, special molecules that signal cells for the regulation of the immune system were released into the blood and made their way to the brain. Already at this point the brain was evaluating what had happened and, in tandem with the chemical input, recruited glucose to get on with the job of addressing the injury and any incoming infection. In addition, a shot of adrenaline (epinephrine) in the blood readied me for action, while noradrenaline readied the brain and other organs to try to restore the status quo. In short, a set of signals, up and down, afferent and efferent, were set in motion to deal with the injury. So far so good, but where is pain in this?

Sensation is not pain, so long as it is without evaluation. Evaluation is also triggered by the injury, but involves all kinds of factors having nothing to do with the nervous system or the brain. My immediate response to the hot poker was a fascinated scrutiny of the changes to my skin, which changed before my eyes (a sense of novelty), followed by fear—not of the injury but of punishment—followed by anxiety, since it was clear that I was going to have to confess to my idiocy immediately, whereupon shame followed in short order. The unpleasantness of the sensation was heightening. Describing what I had done—'I touched the poker'—elicited a response that confirmed alarm, danger, and a painful situation: 'You have *burned* yourself!' Only at this point, and as my hand was thrust under running cold water, accompanied by exclamations concerning my stupidity and about how dangerous my actions were, did the action, the feeling, and the pain coalesce into the reflexive awareness that 'I am *burnt*. It is burning *me*'.

Whatever knowledge we have about the nervous system's response to injury, we cannot call this, by itself, 'a sensation of pain', even though it is extremely difficult to discipline oneself not to do so. The evaluation of injury defines the experience of the pain as pain, beyond mere sensation, and although this is probably processed primarily in the forebrain it is not reducible to the brain's mediation. As University of California neurologist Howard Fields put it, the 'neurobiology of the evaluative component is still an open question'. Perhaps more importantly, we should recognize that not all the answers will be supplied by neurobiology. The experience of my pain depended on a rapid set of reflections and evaluations that were specific to my life and my context. Concerns about having behaved badly, about being punished, about the fragile status of my own pride, and so on, were unique to me in that time and place. No two poker pinchings would be the same.

Contingent pain

The exchange of signals in the spinal cord, between the injury site and the brain, leaves a great amount of room for the cultural context of pain. Indeed, the formulation of the gate control has been the impetus for more holistic studies of situated pain, but with a major limitation: it still depended on nervous stimulation—injury—to talk about pain, its absence, or its modification. It did not effectively account for the enduring suffering of those in chronic pain. It has long puzzled pain scientists why certain things are painful at certain times and places, but not at other times and places. There is a separate set of explanations for the variability of immediate reactions to injury and the fact that even severe trauma may not initially hurt, which I'll come to shortly. But in a more general sense, the brain can respond to a literal or figurative 'rubbing better'.

The gate control theory helped us understand this kind of thing by reference to a set of instructions from the brain to the gate control whether to allow the pain signals through. Experience provides sufficient reassurance that this or that injury is not worthy of our attention and, thus, we do not attend to it. Reassurance, knowledge, experience are salves against pain, 'rubbing it better'. Uncertainty and fear can make pain more acute. This also explains why two identical injuries might cause radically different responses in the same person, depending on where and how they happen. An inoculation jab in a doctor's office, under controlled circumstances and with reassurance, may feel like nothing. A needle prick while attempting to sew a button may sting and cause alarm, exacerbated by the unexpected bleeding. On the other hand, a man with a fear of doctors or of hypodermic needles may be terrified, and thus greatly pained, by the inoculation, but think nothing of a pricked finger if regularly employed as a sempster.

This brings us back to the curious phenomenon of serious injuries that, in the first instance, do not hurt. Henry Beecher (1904–76), a leading light in 20th-century anaesthesiology, wondered how it could be that soldiers suffering severe trauma could claim to be in no serious discomfort. Later, Patrick Wall would observe cases in which accident victims did not feel the pain of crushed or severed limbs until well after the accident. All too commonly, people in serious accidents claim no memory of the incident that maimed them, or at least, no memory of any pain associated with it (even if the long-term consequences of the accident prove to be very painful and persistent). This is, in part, due to a sensory overload that shuts down all possibilities of injury signals reaching the brain.

A more prosaic way of understanding this in humans, however, is to think of it in terms of 'attention'. We only sense pain to which we attend. In the moment of a serious accident, there are pressing concerns that command our attention, not the least of which is 'How do I get out?' This, combined with the rush of adrenalin and the brain's arsenal of built-in pain-relieving chemistry, explains the extraordinary accounts of people who, despite serious injury, manage to carry on with sufficient purpose, bringing themselves or others to safety, before collapsing from their injuries. It is the basis of the marathon runner's focus; of the soldier's imperturbability; of the accident victim's tenacity. Only once the race is over, the battle is done, safety from the crash site is secured—only then does the pain kick in, when we can attend to it and when we perceive the threat of our injuries.

The affective or emotional component of pain, according to these descriptions of contemporary understandings of how pain works, should be eminently clear. As David B. Morris (b. 1942) in *The Culture of Pain* (1991) and Patrick Wall in *Pain* (2000) have both made plain, there is no experience of pain without its affective component. Pain has to *mean* something in order to be experienced as pain at all, and we derive meaning through our affective encounter with something. Hence the meaning of injury in a happy, joyful, or ecstatic context might not be 'pain' per se, and might be completely different from the meaning of an injury in a context of uncertain safety, anxiety, fear, and so on. Unless the affective centres of the brain are actively involved in the physical process of interpreting signals sent from an injury site, there is no pain experience as we would commonly understand it. This has theoretical consequences that are beginning to push the boundaries of what we think of when we think of the circumstances of pain and can be demonstrated through an account of those who cannot experience pain because of congenital analgesia. We must address the possibilities of pain without lesion, and a meaningful re-invigoration of the claim that pain is 'all in the mind'.

The importance of affect

Congenital analgesia, or pain asymbolia, is a genetic condition that renders its 'sufferer' unable to ascribe any meaning to painful states. Careful distinction is required here, because this condition does not imply anaesthesia, or an inability to sense harmful stimuli, but rather an inability to ascribe meaning to such stimuli. Injurious stimuli are perceived plainly as pressure, cutting, cramping, etc., but the person who perceives these things is indifferent to them. Research using neuroimaging techniques such as fMRI has shown that so-called 'pain centres' in the brain do, in fact, 'fire' in these people when given painful stimuli, but their 'affective centres' do not. It is precisely because there is no emotional context to the physical problem that the pain does not register as a problem. Without affect, the sensation of pain does not seem like pain at all.

Perhaps, on first reading, such a condition might be thought a great advantage, but it is actually quite the contrary. Here we alight on the evolutionary purpose of pain. An ongoing pain state is a continual reminder to protect an injury site. Hence the limp with crutches, the arm in a sling, the neck brace, etc. All these devices simply augment what we should want to do in any case: limit movement, pressure, and contact with the injured site, for fear of making the problem worse. Only through such respite do injuries heal. A person with congenital analgesia does not limp when wounded in the leg, and would indifferently go on throwing a ball with a broken arm. This failure to conserve an injury—an affective failure—has the effect of wearing out bones, joints, and muscles at a much greater rate than somebody who could feel pain in a 'normal' way. Pain, to put it in plain terms, keeps us alive. The essential ingredient in making this work is emotion.

If properly perceived, physical pain depends on the normative functioning of the affective cortex of the brain, then to what extent does pain depend on injury at all? While on the one hand, the latest research is fully re-uniting body and mind into a biocultural or biosocial entity, where pain does not reduce to one or the other, and is not removable from its social or cultural context, at the same time new research has opened up important clinical possibilities in the field of pain without lesion, 'emotional pain' and 'social pain'.

Nineteenth-century positivists had always assumed that where pain existed an injury must be present, and if no injury could be found the logical conclusion was an insufficiency in surgical and/or physiological sophistication in order to find it. This cast a heavy shadow across the 20th century. It is the basis of what has been called the 'biomedical' definition of pain, in which 'mental' or 'emotional' pain is cast as unreal. The notion that, perhaps, no physical injury is required for the existence of real pain states was slow to emerge. The alternative thesis, for 19th-century experts and their 20th-century followers, was that pain without physical injury was 'all in the mind'. Into the 20th century, lobotomy was regularly carried out, especially in the US, in order to soothe these troubled heads. Thus, much harm was done in the name of palliative care.

The possibilities opened up by neuroscientific investigation are great. Despite some worthy and necessary scepticism about what we are seeing when we look at an fMRI scan of a brain, there can be no question that parts of the brain related to affective or emotional behaviour are involved in pain states, and that these parts of the brain are identically involved under stimuli that replicate the affective conditions of pain, but which do not involve any physical harm. In other words, the thing that gives pain meaning—that makes pain painful—can be observed in situations where the body is completely uncompromised (Figure 10). It should be understood that this is not a new formulation of a separation of mind and body, but rather an expression of the

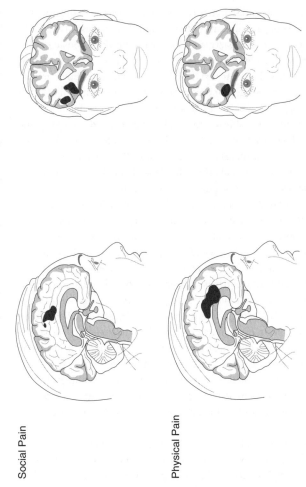

Social Pain

Physical Pain

10. Social and physical pain produce similar brain responses.

physicality of the brain in the body and the effect of non-injurious stimuli on how we feel, physically and emotionally.

Neuroscientific research is returning us full circle to the original concepts of pain in many different global languages. Grief, depression, fear, anxiety, and the like can newly be considered 'painful'. In a now famous test and a series of articles since 2003, Naomi Eisenberger tested the effect of social exclusion among a peer group. Using a computer game of 'cyberball', in which players passed a ball to each other while being scanned, Eisenberger was able to show that being excluded from the game caused brain activity similar to what one would expect to see in conditions of physical pain. Those who felt excluded went through an emotional ordeal that looked, for all intents and purposes, the same as physical pain. The meaning-making processes that are part and parcel of experiencing physical pain appear to be the same when experiencing such things as exclusion, bullying, and grief. A broken heart—the archetype cliché of emotional pain—turns out to be painful in the same sense as a broken leg (although with different consequences, of course). If hurt feelings have been, since time immemorial, a colloquial commonplace, contemporary medicine is beginning to provide a substantial neuroscientific verification of it. While there may not be an exact functional correlation between such social pains and pains arising from physical injury (there are, of course, other factors involved in each case), there is nevertheless a significant functional overlap that suggests the meaningful experience of pain depends on affective brain activity, whether that pain is caused by injury or by grief, broadly construed.

This has general implications for pain killing. Numerous historians have explored the rise of over-the-counter analgesics such as aspirin (acetylsalicylic acid) and paracetamol (acetaminophen). These effective painkillers started life in the first half of the 20th century in the midst of a host of nostrums, taking a detour in the 1950s and 1960s to become alleviators of nervous states in overwhelmed housewives. Those marketing techniques gradually disappeared, challenged as sexist and unsubstantiated. Later, well into the 20th century, these drugs were re-purposed specifically to target physical pain and discomfort, from backache to headaches. Recent studies have newly tested these non-opiate analgesics on 'emotional pain', on the basis that efficacy might be understood as toning down the affective states that give pain meaning. Trials showed that aspirin might well be of significant help for those whose suffering would not have traditionally been defined as pain: the grief stricken, the socially ostracized, and people with existential fears. Indeed, acetaminophen's emotional effects were confirmed by research from Ohio State University in 2015, which found the drug 'blunted' positive as well as negative affective responses to visual stimuli.

Pain killers and placebo

In general, analgesics have proven more effective in cases of emotional pain than placebo, but it is necessary also to pause and reflect on the power of placebo, as it relates to the story of pain. Given what we now know about pain and how to soothe it—a context of reassurance can be a genuinely effective pain reliever—it makes sense that any drug, device, magic word, or physical manipulation might have an analgesic effect, so long as the sufferer believes it will work. Once we understand that the meaning of pain is derived affectively, not from an injury alone, then we can appreciate how any means that might restore our affective cortex to a calm and balanced state would be of benefit. So long as the patient believes the pill, injection, talking cure, massage, stretch, or whatever, will lessen his pain, then in many cases it will. The body contains its own pain-killing system of endogenous opioids, endorphins, dopamine, serotonin, oxytocin, which the body recruits to ward off the signs of pain. The brain's response to painful situations, physical and emotional, is to trigger these chemical cascades. The administration of certain analgesic drugs can be understood not so much as the introduction of exogenous painkillers, but rather as the enhancement of the body's own endogenous pain-killing system.

Acetaminophen is thought to work in precisely this fashion. Through a series of chemical processes within the spinal cord, acetaminophen indirectly inhibits the body's capacity to process an endogenous cannabinoid called anandamide. The endocannabinoid system in the body helps regulate memory, appetite, and metabolism, and cannabinoids are recruited as modulators of noradrenaline in painful situations. After the administration of a placebo, it is the endocannabinoid system that causes the painkilling effect. After the administration of acetaminophen, the body boosts the production of anandamide in the central nervous system, causing a diminution of the spinal cord's capacity to detect pain. In other words, when you take a Tylenol or a paracetamol, you are in effect kick-starting your own central nervous system to produce more of its own painkillers.

Cutting-edge research from Harvard Medical School's Program in Placebo Studies has recently pointed to the possibility of a genetic network in neurotransmitter (dopamine, serotonin, etc.) pathways that effects the extent to which an individual responds to placebo, and the extent to which drugs and placebos might act on one another. This apparent genetic variability suggests a weakness in the common model of controlled trials, in which drug performance is rated against placebo performance, and indeed the Harvard scholars call for the introduction of a 'no-treatment control' in clinical trials as a check against placebo–drug interaction.

These genetic discoveries are compounded by cultural studies that also point to the vagaries of placebo as control in clinical trials. A recent study headed by Jeffrey Mogil at McGill University found that, in the United States at least, the placebo effect appears to be on the rise. Pharmaceutical companies who want to launch new pain-killing drugs to the market have first to pass strictly controlled trials in which the new drug has to outperform the placebo effect. Increasingly, it is becoming difficult to beat the body's own analgesic system, and the vast majority of new drugs fail to reach the market. Why? That is uncertain, but a number of speculations have arisen that may in turn prove to be of great advantage to those who find themselves in pain in a clinical setting. The first theory is that the particular cultural practice, especially in the US, of television advertising of pharmaceuticals to a consumer market has created an overwhelming sense of awe at the power of new drugs. Entering into a trial predisposed culturally to expect drugs to do wonders might lead to a powerful placebo effect. Other theories point to the size, duration, and staging of American trials, which tend to employ larger samples, longer trial times, and grand presentations. When trial participants are initially impressed by the magnitude of investment, even aesthetically, they are more likely to respond positively to placebo. It has been pointed out that American trials often employ nurses whose only task is to administer to trial participants. The disposition of medical practitioners is well known to have a correlative effect on the pain of patients, and in lavish trials this probably also plays into the heightened placebo response.

While this leaves pharmaceutical companies scratching their heads about how to get a drug through testing and onto the market, it also foregrounds an opportunity to make the lives of people in pain better in the clinical setting. Happy nurses, friendly, confident doctors, and a sense of lavish expense in the hospital or surgery environment may well diminish pain. Whatever it is that drug companies do in American pain-killer trials to elicit such a high degree of placebo response might be replicated in the 'real' world. Most importantly, a new set of proofs of the biopsychosocial nature of pain experience opens up new possibilities for the largest group of people in pain, those for whom pain is considered a syndrome: those in chronic pain.

Chapter 8
Chronic pain

The scope of the problem

Marcus Aurelius (121–180 CE), Roman Emperor and Stoic philosopher in his own right, understood something about pain that has only recently been explored in any depth. Intolerable pain resulted in death, so he thought, but the pain which 'holds long must needs be tolerable'. The sufferer of chronic pain has to find ways to avert the attention of the mind from the trouble in order to endure. The specific term for pain that 'holds long' in Marcus Aurelius' *Meditations* maps onto the concept of labour or toil, just as we have seen in Genesis. As a metaphor for chronic pain, nothing could be more apt.

Insofar as chronic pain has been the purview of institutions of medicine, it is a relatively young phenomenon, having come to light in a major way after the carnage of the First World War. Other global conflicts throughout the 20th century, in combination with perceived breakdowns in social communities and family life, have exacerbated the problem. What constitutes the distinction between acute and chronic pain in terms of time is somewhat arbitrary, but it is normally considered to involve pain lasting at least three months. Pain that endures is associated with many conditions, from sciatica to arthritis to multiple sclerosis, and is experienced in a variety of ways, from unremitting burning to unrelenting aches. It is a massive medical and social problem, the scale of which has proven difficult to measure due to the vagaries of definitions and surveys. Nonetheless, studies for the United Kingdom have found that anywhere between 11.5 and 35 per cent of adults experience chronic pain. In Canada the number is as high as 44 per cent. In Australia, anywhere between 18 and 50 per cent.

Although a conception of chronic pain is as old as concepts of pain itself, sufferers of chronic pain in particular have been victims of the dualistic separation of physical and mental pain in modernity. Medical focus in the 20th century on physical injury (lesion) as the principal reliable indication of pain put many chronic sufferers at a disadvantage. In the first place, chronic pain sufferers often cannot point to, or prove, the presence of an injury. The countless millions of low-back pain sufferers will attest to this. Only a small minority of them can demonstrate clearly the cause of their complaint. Many of the rest go untreated or undertreated, not necessarily because there is a lack of treatment options available, but because of a lack of access to such treatments through ordinary medical and clinical channels. Other sufferers might once have been able to point to an injury, but after the acute phase is over and the injury healed, the pain is supposed to go away. What if it doesn't?

Chronic sufferers have battled compassion fatigue among their friends and family, and, historically, a suspicion of malingering among the medical community. Worse still, they are party to the suspicions. What if it's all in my head? Shouldn't I just be able to shake this off? And then, when the pain remains, it is augmented by guilt, shame, and self-loathing, as well as depression, isolation, self-medication, and an increased likelihood of suicide or suicide ideation. A recent Australian study found that the chance of 'suicidality' was two to three times greater in chronic pain sufferers, and that two-thirds of those who attempted suicide over a twelve-month period (2006–7) suffered from chronic pain.

Severe chronic pain has been shown to have a close association with increased mortality risk, especially from heart and respiratory disease. Public health ethicists in the US, Daniel Goldberg among them, have decried the almost overwhelming evidence of the under-treatment (and under-reporting) of pain in that country, and the massive effort of will, policy reform, and education, both of doctors and patients, required to change this state of affairs. In part this is in response to a 2011 Institute of Medicine report, which estimated 116 million adults in the US experience chronic pain. Of these, some fifty million are partly or wholly disabled by it.

The chronic pain anomaly

If we return to the IASP's official definition of pain, we can begin to understand the anomaly of chronic pain. The definition makes explicit that pain is 'associated with actual or potential tissue damage, or described in terms of such damage'. What if there is no such damage or potential for it? What if it cannot be so described? As we have seen, it was only in the late 20th century that pain expressions were medically grouped according to a predefined and limited range of possibilities. Sufferers of chronic pain in particular may often feel silenced by the range of permissible metaphors available to them. Elaine Scarry (b. 1946), who argued forcefully and persuasively that pain is world destroying, silencing, uncommunicable, gives credence to such fears. Chronic pain sufferers, especially in the 20th century, when new and innovative ways of hurting were coupled with new and innovative ways of preserving, have struggled to find words to describe their pain that fit the descriptions that medical personnel had been trained to hear and to acknowledge as idiomatic descriptions of pain. When a person's pain experience does not fit with medical paradigms of injury and tissue damage, does that make the pain any the less real to the subject? Such pain may not be divisible into physical signs and/or psychological pathology. 'Pain' itself may not be an adequate word, or concept, for what sufferers endure. It has often been stated that there is not an adequate word, and there are not adequate institutions, for sufferers of chronic pain.

With acute pain, usually associated with injury, straightforward explanations of its evolutionary purpose have sufficed to authenticate the experience of it. Chronic pain seems to be categorically different. While a person's pain may have had an initial acute cause, it is by no means necessary of all cases of chronic pain. Moreover, the ongoing suffering of chronic pain can be out of all proportion to an initial injury, and persists even after the injury is healed. In short, many sufferers of chronic pain have no specific physical damage that accounts for their misery. Chronic pain is not a warning to withdraw; it does not assist in the healing process; it appears to have no evolutionary purpose.

Chronic pain therefore presents a significant functional mystery to be cracked. If not a 'warning' that compels you to pull your foot from the fire or, when suffering from a burnt foot, a reminder to keep it from being touched or bearing weight, what is it? Many of the chemical cascades that flow through the nervous system in painful situations are known to be a response to 'threat', which might actually be the presence of an injury or it might be a threat in the more typical sense of something that primes us to fight or flee, or roots us to the spot in helplessness. One potential explanation for the unrelenting suffering in chronic pain states is a failure in the internal systems that recognize threat. In that sense, chronic pain can again be placed under the 'warning' rubric of pain usefulness, with the caveat that the warning system is fundamentally broken. Understanding the nature of that breakage has entailed the generation of a new theory of how individuals conceive of themselves as bodies, and with it a new multidimensional understanding of pain. Therefore, research into chronic pain now works on the premise that it is a disease in its own right. Promising enquiries are orientated around the assumption that, for the person in chronic pain, something must be going wrong. If there is no injury, there must nevertheless be some pathology of the nervous system or the brain. The goal, unlike with acute pains that help keep us alive, is to eliminate it.

Phantom pain

Phantom limb pain—an enduring pain that emanates from a part of the body that no longer exists—has activated more research in this direction than anything else. Many people think that phantom pain might be the key to understanding and to treating chronic pain more generally, especially where there are no clear pathological causes. Knowledge of phantom pain has been around for hundreds of years. French surgeon Ambroise Paré (1510–90) mentioned the phenomenon in 1552; René Descartes described it in 1641. But serious applied thinking about phantoms really only arose in the late 19th century, with Silas Weir Mitchell's (1829–1914) studies of phantom limbs in the American Civil War. The dramatic increase in numbers of youthful amputees in 20th-century warfare furnished many more cases. Improvements in field surgery had ensured that many of the injured in battle survived, only to re-adjust with difficulty to civilian life.

A large, but diffuse, community of amputees struggled with stump pain and phantom limb pain. Each individual, generally isolated from others in the same boat, and treated in isolation also, went through a struggle not merely with their own pain but also with the institutions of medicine that could not or would not acknowledge that the pain was real. Individual cases that have been reconstructed by historians tend to show a lack of patience on behalf of medical carers for the difficult plight of the amputee. Phantom pain and stump pain was poorly, if at all, understood, and the continual complaining of the patient was often attributed to flaws of moral character, a lack of 'pluck' or courage, or even a link to sexual 'inversions' (in a time where homosexuality could be conflated with mental illness). Phantom pains and pains without lesion were dismissed as 'all in the mind', indicators of psychological disturbance, and heightened sensitivity. Pains that were all too real to the sufferer could be subsumed under the rubric of 'nervous illness', 'shell shock', 'hysteria', or later 'post-traumatic stress'.

While post-trauma issues certainly did play a large role in the post-war lives of the maimed, these psychological effects were also poorly understood for much of the 20th century. To have the physiological reality of phantom pain treated as a psychogenic problem often made things worse for the individual in pain. For generations, the burden of proving that their pain was real fell on the sufferers themselves, against an entrenched paradigm that only really recognized physical signs of injury. Failure to prove that pain was real led to prescriptions of knuckling down and getting on with things.

A hundred years after the First World War, we still do not have a complete explanation for phantom pain, though there are many theories. Melzack in particular has elaborated on the apparent weaknesses in his own 'gate control theory' to try to account for the mystery of chronic pain, particularly in cases of phantom pain. In published papers between 1989 and 2005, Melzack proposed and maintained a theory of the 'neuromatrix'. Key to this theory is the insistence that experience is not present anywhere, but is created in the neuroplastic brain. Pain is *output* of the brain, not *input* from the periphery. To put it another way, focusing on the site of an (old) injury will not yield insights into the reason for it being enduringly painful. Melzack forcefully states that injury is not pain. Pain is a quality produced in the brain, and is not reconcilable with, or reducible to, injury per se. So much has been recognized since Beecher's observation in the Second World War, that more than two-thirds of seriously injured soldiers reported no pain immediately after having been returned behind the lines for treatment. Patrick Wall noted the same of Israeli soldiers who had suffered traumatic amputations in the Yom Kippur War in 1973. Whatever the arrangement of nerves in the periphery of the body, the experience of pain does not intrinsically inhere in them when damaged. Just as peripheral nerve damage could not account for the absences of pain in injured soldiers, so such damage could not account for the enduring phantom pains of the amputee.

The general shift in direction away from the periphery and the site of the injury to the brain has enabled pain specialists to approach the problem anew. The neuromatrix theory posits the production of a neurosignature of the whole body: an internal neuro 'image' or 'pattern' of the body understood as the self. Melzack conceives of this neurosignature as an experience maker that responds to the barrage of sensory 'inputs' that are particularly heightened at times of injury coming in from the periphery. While the particulars of an individual's neuromatrix may be genetically programmed, it is nevertheless plastic, being formed and informed by a number of factors that together produce a dynamic sense of the self: sensory inputs, including aural and visual, are components; affective and emotional states, which are themselves forged in the crucible of society and culture, play a part; the meanings and values attached to body parts, proportions, postures, and movements—some of them instinctive, some of them socially and culturally prescribed—are factored in. All these inputs are processed and, in Melzack's analogy, 'arranged' into a symphonic output that equates to the body-self. A cut in the leg may or may not be painful, but I know it is a cut in *my* leg because of the neurosignature imprint of my neuromatrix. The neuromatrix promises the collapse of both Cartesian dualism and the distance between biomedicine and phenomenology.

If all experience is produced in the brain, and not intrinsic to anything 'in the world', then we can begin to understand how a missing limb might still be experienced as present. In Melzack's terms, one might put it like this: riding a bike is not the experience of cycling. The experience is only in the brain, processed according to a variety of physiological, psychological, and socio-cultural interpretations of what it *means* and how it *feels* to ride a bike. If one sets out to ride a bike, the movements and postures involved are commanded from the brain, via the nervous system, to the muscles recruited for the task. The 'output' of the neuromatrix that sets off these movements is also processed in the brain to make experience. Since both movement and experience have the neuromatrix in common, it is possible for the original commands and the experience to take place, even if there is no worldly possibility of riding a bike. Amputees who experience phantom limbs have testified precisely to this experience, as if missing legs are pedalling, with the accompanying feelings of tiredness that follow from a prolonged physical activity. As Melzack points out, 'feeling' tired is not a result of sensory input from particular muscles, but rather a result of 'the signature of a neuromodule' recruited for the task of riding. Amputated legs suffer from cycling fatigue because the experience of fatigue in the neuromatrix exists irrespective of the absence of legs.

The explanation for pain in phantom limbs follows on accordingly. The neurosignature 'expects' signals from the limb (it is genetically predisposed to compute the whole body) that do not arrive. The neurosignature response to the cutting of the signal is a pattern of nervous activation that is *experienced* as burning pain. Since the missing limb is part of the body-self neurosignature, no amount of time passed since the loss of the limb will make any difference to this neurological response to the missing modulating signals from the periphery. Similarly, neuromatrix commands to the missing limb to move are increasingly amplified as a result of having no effect, which may result in the *experience* of muscle cramp. All these types of pain are thought to be a result of brain output, rather than caused by the site of the original injury.

Not everyone agrees with this. A debate took place in the journal *Pain* in 2014 among phantom-pain researchers, after Marshall Devor and his team published a paper demonstrating that phantom pain was indeed caused by signals from the peripheral nervous system, not in the amputee's stump, but in the dorsal root ganglia. Questioning about methods and long-term results has yielded no final answer to the question, 'Is it all resolved?', but research continues in which both neuroplasticity and erroneous signalling from the periphery are in play.

New directions

What does this all mean for the future of alleviating phantom limb pain, and chronic pain more generally? Whatever the finer points of the debate on phantom pain, there is general agreement that chronic pain is impossible to understand without a thorough appraisal of affective and socio-cultural elements, fully integrated into a functional definition of pain. In a remarkable transformation of medico-scientific understandings of pain, and with a renewal of hope among many sufferers, chronic pain management increasingly involves a comprehensive understanding of the world—social, emotional, familial, professional—in which the pain is taking place. Though increasingly highly formalized, it is in essence an acknowledgement of historical colloquial knowledge about how people in enduring pain feel. That word, *feel*, remains operative because it encapsulates not only sensation but also emotion, cognition, and, importantly, communication. How a sufferer feels at any point in time is directly related to the degree to which she is able to tell someone how she feels, and the extent to which she is confident that anybody is listening.

Crucially, neuroscientists have recognized that social and emotional factors have a direct bearing on the physiological condition of the body, or rather, that bodies exist within the world. Being in pain comes with associated stress, which has in turn a physiological reaction (physiological stress is also activated by physical injury). Cortisol is the body's own hormonal response to pain. In acute, stressful situations, cortisol is actively useful in increasing blood sugar and stimulating the metabolism. Prolonged production of cortisol in response to lasting stress can have a number of negative effects. The immune system is suppressed. Muscles start to atrophy. Bone and nerve tissue

Pain

degenerates. The combined result can be experienced as more pain, causing further stress, leading to prolonged production of cortisol, and so on. The body, the world around it (its context), and the mind are a pain-making whole. Anger, anxiety, and depression are therefore highly correlated with the under-treatment of chronic pain. The isolated chronic pain sufferer can be thought of as being in compound pain, complete with an internal spiralling logic of despair. That despair tends to be highly personalized, relating to the sufferer's own context of profession, family, community, medical history, self-image, location, and so on.

To break the cycle, one must interrupt the production of stress (both psychological and physiological). Since many of the symptoms of chronic pain are exacerbated by isolation and feelings of exclusion from the medical system, one possible step is to provide meaningful and supportive company, and actively make the medical system more transparently open to chronic pain sufferers. Even where the root cause of the pain is still unknown, social support tailored to the individual case is likely to be a salve to some extent. Research has shown that social support can alleviate social pain, or even prevent it being triggered in the first place. Since chronic pain is so intimately bound up with social isolation and self-recrimination, finding social means to alleviate these problems should be helpful in clearing some of the painful fog of chronic pain. In addition, it has been demonstrated that drugs developed as anti-depressants can have a positive effect on the alleviation of some types of chronic pain. Given the high degree of neural overlap between emotional maladies and the experience of pain, it is unsurprising that there is cross-over impact with this kind of drug.

To a similar end, mindfulness research has found that meditative practices that focus on emotional control can effectively alter pain experience by reducing pain anticipation and by neutralizing emotional appraisals of sensation. Technological innovation similarly exploits brain plasticity. Early successes with purposeful control of parts of the brain that are particularly associated with physical signs of pain, under the guidance of real-time fMRI feedback, suggest both the possibilities for pain management and the extent to which socio-technological innovations can materially change what is happening in the brain and at the level of experience. Technological advances come with the promise of reflexive auto-control of brain output: perhaps pain experience can be effectively self-modulated under directed training.

Another insight has been to identify people who are predisposed to fears of illness or injury or who are susceptible to anxiety. Where individuals first come into contact with medicine—after a car crash, perhaps, or when diagnosed with shingles—their personality traits can be investigated to determine the probability that their initial injury or illness is likely to develop into a chronic pain syndrome. For these people, and for people already in chronic pain, a programme of fear and anxiety reduction has been shown to have a measurable positive impact on quality of life. Moreover, while there may be some genetic conditions that make some people more likely to suffer chronic pain than others, a general awareness of the situated causes of fear, anger, and anxiety should help to make it easier to alleviate suffering as and when it occurs. These are social and cultural factors that go beyond asking simple questions about an individual's employment, family, lifestyle, pressures, and intentions. Rather, they get at the construction of emotions themselves: the objects of fear, anxiety, and anger are not universal, even if the human stress system and the damaging effects of long-term exposure to cortisol are. Hospitals, doctors, medical instruments, drugs, social services, medical insurance, and personal appearance are all, to some extent, implicated as objects of fear, anxiety, and anger themselves. The structure, administration, personnel, and location of chronic pain management therefore have to be taken into account in contemporary approaches to address the emotional aspects of chronic pain.

Chapter 9
Cultures of pain

Pain as a process

Pain, as will be evident by now, is never *just* pain. Objective
measurements, biological universals, and timeless standards:
all attempts to find the key to how pain works have failed to
describe how pain feels, precisely because pain experience is in
the world and made by minds. How it is expressed and how it is
felt are in a dynamic relationship with the body (including the
mind) in society and culture. The biocultural and psychosocial
phenomenon of pain experience takes place, by very definition,
in a context of social and cultural prescriptions and proscriptions,
affirmations and denials. The veracity of a pain experience
depends on the capacity and willingness of witnesses to pain to
identify this experience as painful. Where pain is denied, dismissed,
discounted, sufferers struggle to find words and meanings for
what is happening to them. Perhaps, in their struggle, they change
the cultural context of pain in order to gain recognition or
validation for their pain. To effect such change might involve
uniting a community of sufferers (now increasingly possible, over
great distances, thanks to social media) in order to give substance
to individual voices. Perhaps they subscribe to the dominant view,
and knuckle down and carry on regardless. Likewise, this depends
on subscription to a community view. In between, sufferers might
struggle, not knowing how to feel about whatever is bothering

them. Perhaps fear of the unknown makes their complaint more acute. Perhaps a discourse of reassurance reduces the suffering.

In all of these cases, the defining characteristic of biocultural pain experience is that it is a process. Individuals work out, through the range of expressions and bodily practices available to them in their specific culture, how they feel, trying to give voice or movement to what hurts but doesn't speak for itself. In turn, the process of matching a felt pain state to an available pain expression, alters the pain state itself. This process can be seen at work in many cultures of pain, and is the decisive interpretive tool for working out why pain and its accompanying politics seem to change over time, and from place to place. At the extreme end of this process, where a pain state is completely denied by its witnesses, to the dismay of the sufferer, a crisis may set in. In such conditions, there is no way to put the pain experience into the world and, as Elaine Scarry famously said of the victims of torture in *The Body in Pain* (1985), the world around this person collapses.

Clearly it would be a mistake to think that, all things being equal, pain cannot be effectively communicated. The experience of pain is dependent not only on the complexities of the nervous system, and the descending regulatory chemistry of the brain, but also on one's past experience, and on one's social and cultural environment. In a context where certain injuries are ritually inflicted—rites of passage surrounded by a rhetoric of reassurance or even celebration—these injuries may not only be readily understood; they may not even hurt. Hence the famous Hindu Chidi Mari 'hook swinging' festival documented by Melzack and Wall in *The Challenge of Pain* (1982), in which a 'celebrant' hangs from ropes attached to steel hooks that pierce the flesh of the back, apparently without pain.

The opposite holds true: in rites of passage or rituals that reinforce power dynamics of gender, class, or caste, and which take place in an atmosphere of fear and/or lack of complicity, as in the case of female genital mutilation, for example, the pain can be substantial. Then again, in many rituals, pain is considered to be a necessary part of transformation, when the intensity of the pain is correlated to meaningfulness, both for the individual and for the group. Bioarchaeologists like Pamela Gellar have argued that the pain associated with ritual modification of teeth among pre-Colombian Maya was central to a shared experience of identity transformation into adulthood and seemed to embody social identification. An individual may reconcile himself to what looks from the outside to be a painful ordeal to the point that the pain is accepted as necessary or dismissed.

How this contextual variation in pain experience works has seemed mysterious, but one of the important consequences of recent neuroscientific work on pain has been to shed light on how cultural context might directly affect the experience of pain. The more deeply researchers delve into the brain, the more they are turning to a biocultural understanding of brain functioning. What happens to the body and mind in a pain state is always mediated through the broad social context of the sufferer. In short, no amount of searching in the brain and central nervous system alone is going to lead to a definitive answer to what pain is and how it works. Our brains and our bodies are plastic; they are to some degree writeable objects. Often, the cultural inscriptions are beyond individual control, though they are not beyond analysis. Proof of the cultural element of pain comes from all quarters. The historian can easily point to the vast array of different pain expressions and experiences to demonstrate that being in pain has been far from constant. But while historical knowledge might have once seemed anecdotal, recent technological and sociological research has provided more measurable data on the contingencies of pain experience.

One of the most striking observations to come from the neuroimaging world, mentioned briefly in Chapter 8, is that brain function can be honed, practiced, and controlled through targeted training in real-time fMRI scanners. Briefly, test subjects were shown to be able, through feedback about real-time scanning of their own brains, to activate targeted sections of the brain related to particular motor functions while, in fact, they were only imagining the movements that the brain activity normally represented. Essentially, a new technology enables human beings to, quite literally, control areas of their own brains. Such training implies many new possibilities for human experience. Since emotions are integral to all pain experiences, whether related to injury, pathology, or otherwise, the capacity to self-regulate neural activity in affective centres of the brain—in essence, introducing autonomy to automatic systems—suggests new vistas for pain management. Significantly, these vistas depend on access to new techniques and technologies: objects of material culture have the capacity to redefine the experience of (especially chronic) pain. A greater recognition of the importance of social and cultural factors in the modification of pain experience is being complemented by technologies that potentially harness cultural modifiers so as to put pain relief in the hands—the minds—of sufferers. New methods of seeing and sharing pain—and therefore new methods of modifying pain—are on the horizon.

Practices of sharing pain

However varied our pain experiences have been over time and place, these experiences have always been related to the manner in which they were shared. Sharing pain is partly about language, but the words we use are only an epiphenomenon of a much broader array of gestures and utterances we use to signify our plight to others in ways they will understand. The qualification 'ways they will understand' is essential to our ability to analyse the social and cultural aspects of pain and pain experience. The history of hysteria makes for an illustrative case.

Up until the early 19th century, a patient presenting with a rigidly arched back, gritted teeth, and clenched fists and toes would be presumed either to have tetanus or to be demonically possessed. A whole range of artistic representations of the latter can be found from the Renaissance onwards. When, in the 1800s, Charles Bell (1774–1842) set about making pictorial representations of human physical expressions more accurate, a cross-over of artistic technique and anatomical investigation, he found some key markers to distinguish the true sufferer of tetanus—an extremely painful condition—and those who were, to him, obviously faking (Figure 11). In the budding era of scientific and medical rationalism there was little room for any entertainment of demons, which had the effect of relegating the possessed to the realms of mania, melancholia, hypochondria, and, most significantly, hysteria. All of these labels had, at some point or other, some basis in a physical ailment, but in the 19th century they came to refer to ailments of the mind that were detectable through the non-pathological physical presentations of the body.

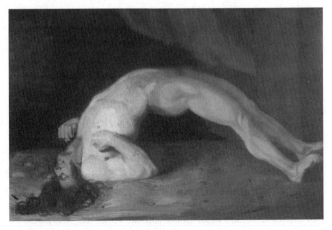

11. Charles Bell, *Opisthotonos* (1809).

If Bell had exposed the hysterical tetanus arch as fraud, he also set in motion the cultural possibility for a uniformly understood physical expression of hysterical pain. The status of that pain was contested. We might now readily subsume hysterical pain under the widening rubric of depression or anxiety, and, with what we know about the neurological reality of emotional pain, take it seriously *as* pain. Nineteenth-century doctors were not necessarily so open to taking hysteria seriously as bona fide suffering, whether considered as a syndrome or a pathology. When the Parisian neurologist Jean-Martin Charcot undertook his now legendary study of hysterical patients at the *Salpêtrière* in Paris, in the last decades of the 19th century, he quickly stumbled upon the startling reality that all of his hysterics presented this *faux*-tetanus arch very soon after having been admitted to his care.

It has since been demonstrated that the expression, which Charcot mistook for a classic and reliable indication of hysteria, was effectively taught to the patients by Charcot himself, along with his staff. Hysterical patients were unconsciously coached to behave in a way that could be understood, classified, and then treated. The sense of reward garnered from so behaving no doubt assisted the patients on their roads to recovery. This is not to say that the patients consciously faked the posture of hysterical pain. On the contrary, all the evidence points to the power of suggestion and the need to find a bodily expression for emotional suffering that would make sense to the audience with whom it was shared. These were not performative acts in the theatrical sense (whatever Charcot's own sense of the theatrical), but emotive acts. Pain—even where it was essentially written off as hysteria—was shared through signs and utterances that could be readily received, interpreted, and acted upon by witnesses to pain. In our lives we may never have cause to resort to such postures, but all of our expressions have to 'fit' in the context where they will be correctly understood.

News of Charcot's discovery quickly made it into the consciousness of a broad swathe of society. Women across Europe and extending even to Europe's imperial outposts suddenly came down with readily identifiable cases of hysteria, replete with the hysterical arch, but with no lasting signs of actual tetanus. While diagnosis might have come with a prescription for moral or sexual reform from doctors, the hysterical arch was doubtless an effective form of communication of pain among a community of women. Its apparently high degree of contagion suggests that women (and some men) were precisely in need of a bodily sign of their social and emotional pain.

We can be sure of the socio-cultural influence here because the hysterical arch, once so common, is now rarely seen. After the discovery of the tetanus bacterium in 1897 and the shift in tetanus diagnosis from one of posture to one of infection, the hysterical arch quickly disappeared from everyday medical experience. The capacity to vaccinate against tetanus (available from 1924) made spurious cases of the disease less likely, and indeed they became much less common. In other words, once the specificities of the disease were established as being pathological, rather than merely postural, the effectiveness of the posture as a sign of pain became less plausible. Hysterics, increasingly being otherwise defined as 'shell shocked' or 'nervous', found other means of communicating their pain.

This brief sketch shows the contingency intrinsic to the biopsychosocial model of pain. Contemporary pain management generally takes social factors into account, from daily activities to interpersonal relations, and from social expectations to work history, but there is not yet a rigorous method of weighing the relative importance of each factor, or of assessing the extent to which those factors might change. In the narrative offered here, of hysterics finding a common posture to express their emotional pain (which was nevertheless dismissed as chicanery by the medical community), social expectations were of primary importance. Doubtless, however, few of the patients who presented with the hysterical arch could have articulated those expectations, and there is no evidence that patients consciously knew what they were doing. To assess the impact of social expectations and other social and cultural factors in the experience and expression of pain, therefore, we have to step back and ask fundamental questions about our own cultural assumptions.

When the leading American pain specialist, John Bonica, was sent to explore the possibilities and science behind traditional Chinese medicine in the 1970s, for example, there was an urge to overwrite Chinese cultural practices with Western medical rationales. Acupuncture in Mao's (1893–1976) China clearly worked for a lot of people a lot of the time, but also seemed to depend to a large extent on cultural beliefs about its efficacy. American doctors tried to reduce it to its underlying physiological mechanisms, postulating that perhaps acupuncture served to 'close the gate', and therefore block pain, thus lending weight to both the 'gate control' theory and the physiological efficacy of acupuncture as an anaesthetic. But in the final analysis, American doctors who visited China (Patrick Wall had also gone on an exploratory visit) dismissed Chinese explanations about acupuncture's influence on the body's energy flows, concluding that it was in effect a form of hypnotism. We know now from great experience that many medicines and pain-relieving practices work because of a placebo effect. That effect, as we have seen, can be scientifically researched, but what causes the effect seems to be infinitely variable. Just as, for the women of the late 19th century who found expression for their anguish in the hysterical arch, so the believer in alternative medicine may derive some pain relief from it in some cases, even if it can be conclusively demonstrated to have no intrinsic chemical or physiological efficacy beyond placebo.

Figures of pain

Finding expression for pain, as we have seen, is far from limited to linguistic constructions. We do not only talk about pain, but embody it and project it. While many of the medical attempts to try to understand pain through metaphor have focused on what is being done to the body—it is being pierced, cramped, stabbed, shot—those who endure pain have often tried to make less concrete statements about what it feels like to experience their own pain. This often defies language. Serbian artist Mladen Stilinović (b. 1947) captured the problem, but also transcended it, with his 2000–3 work, *Dictionary—Pain*, with each page of the dictionary individually framed and with every single entry's definition replaced with the single word 'pain'. Photographer Deborah Padfield found, by co-producing photographs of pain with pain patients at University College Hospital in London, that images were 're-invigorating existing language, initiating a symbiotic relationship between words and images capable of generating new language'. Giving patients agency in the production of pain material allowed them a feeling of ownership of their own pain and a new medium of validation in the clinical setting. These are both ways of putting pain into the world and making it available, to the self and others.

Friedrich Nietzsche (1844–1900), German philosopher and lifelong sufferer of ill health and chronic pain, employed a similar strategy by naming his pain 'dog', remarking on its fidelity, lack of shame, and its wisdom. The inner beast, which he scolded like a chattel, hardly fits any medical scheme, but it likely makes sense to anyone who has chronically suffered. Looking at Nietzsche's death mask in an exhibition on pain in art in Berlin (Hamburger Bahnhof, 2007), one could not help but search the immortalized knitted brow for the traces of canine pain. What is in this face of immortalized pain that also signifies its eternal cessation? We can but wonder. When I first encountered this object, accompanied as it was by Nietzsche's description of his pain animal, I could not help but project my own appreciation of suffering into it. I 'empathized', to use the word in a technical and aesthetic sense, with this dead, inorganic, material object. To be sure, Nietzsche's death mask is not Nietzsche, but it is somehow a capturing of Nietzsche's pain (Figure 12).

Pain is a major theme in the world of art, and it succeeds and perpetuates precisely because it manages to project outwards in non-linguistic terms what it feels like to be in pain. The history of art offers a rich seam of evidence to mine for the ways in which expressive contexts and the reception of pain have transformed. Popular depictions of the experience of pain defy description, precisely because the image outperforms words. The massive range of styles and expressions speaks to the equivocity of pain, its mutability and contextual contingency, while at the same time pointing to a constant category. That category, as Joan Scott (b. 1941) once said of gender, is at once empty and overflowing. It has no transcendent form or content, yet we all fill it with meanings such that we can understand each other's pain, or sometimes so that we can communicate that our pain is not understood.

Francis Bacon (1909–92), in particular, was a master of articulating the unsayable; of finding an outlet for human pain and suffering that goes beyond the possibilities of linguistic construction. He obliterates the human body and demonstrates its close connection to mere butchered meat, while at the same time elevating an experience of suffering—of *passion*, in an old-fashioned sense—as something distinctly and irrevocably human. His *Three Studies for a Crucifixion* (1962), for example, conflates the wracked body and spiritual agony, joining the human of modernity to the Western exemplar of suffering: Christ (Figure 13). It is impossible adequately to describe the way that these contorted bodies and carcasses embody or express

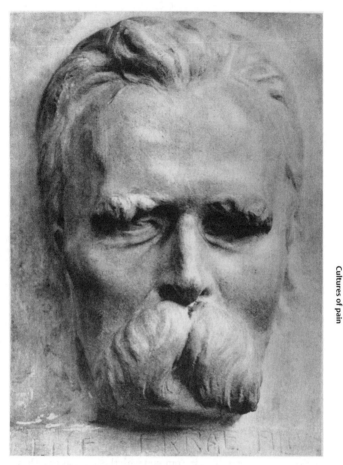

12. Rudolf Saudek, *Death Mask of Nietzsche* (*c.*1910).

their pain, but the fact that they do so is inescapable, even to the untrained eye. They encompass grief, loss, suffering, injury, and anguish, wrapping them up into one entangled and complex, but readily accessible expression of what, for want of a better word, we call pain.

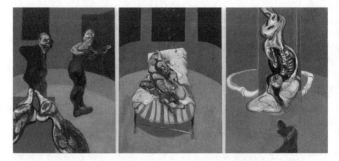

13. Francis Bacon, *Three Studies for a Crucifixion* (1962).

Readily accessible? For some of us, perhaps, and for now. If Bacon's expressions of pain show us anything, however, it is that the community of understanding is both geographically and historically limited (Figure 13). Imagine a Victorian art critic poring over Bacon's canvasses. Imagine, moreover, Victorian sufferers having easy access to these images. What would they make of them, save for blasphemy and obscenity? What will future onlookers see and feel when exposed to past iterations of suffering? What does a sufferer from outside of the Judeo-Christian tradition make of the allusions and illusions in what essentially apes the altarpiece triptych? As with the example of the grieving faces in the depiction of Christ as Man of Sorrows, a general sense of the continuity of expressions of pain only gets us so far. To reach a fuller understanding requires a literacy of cultural signs and symbols, as well as an appreciation of the context in which expressions of pain are made. To this extent, art historical analysis shares something in common with the latest approaches to pain management.

The vicissitudes of experience

Critical reflexivity is becoming much more important to the clinical setting, where a person in pain meets medical personnel. The respective epistemologies brought to bear in this situation may not necessarily be commensurate with each other. The vernacular epistemology of the patient, with her colloquial understanding of what hurts, how it feels, and how to express this feeling, is met by the expert, specialist, and professional epistemology of the physician or nurse. The latter may focus only in part on what the patient says but probe in different ways, through tests, physical examination, and experience to get to a diagnosis. Experience, in this case, refers not only to the hours logged personally consulting with patients, but also to the repertoire of knowledge and its accompanying practices that are passed down through medical education as a professional orthodoxy of approach.

This, in turn, is bounded by suspicion. Western doctors in particular carry instilled concerns about the perils of drug dependency when prescribing opioids to patients in pain. Such fears were dismissed by Melzack and Wall decades ago, but inefficiencies in prescription management and control have led to a rising tide of media coverage about the tragedies of prescription-drug addiction. Doctors are therefore guarded against the prescription or administration of narcotics. There is also still a tendency to maintain, despite the weight of evidence against a mind-body duality, a learnt proclivity to divide up patient pain into 'real' (i.e. having a mechanical cause) and 'psychogenic' (i.e. existing only as a form of mental illness). On top of these things, medical personnel are inevitably culturally situated, and may unconsciously bring to bear assumptions about gender, age, and ethnicity, and their respective relationships to pain sensitivity and tolerance. Sometimes these combined factors lead to over-medication and/or greater amounts of attention. Sometimes they have the opposite effect.

The patient, meanwhile, feels a certain pressure to convince the doctor or nurse of the reality of her pain. This involves a level of performance that privileges the educated, who might better speak the language of medicine. The patient may also encounter a complex emotional barrage when faced with medical settings: fear (of what might be wrong, and/or of being dismissed); guilt (about taking up the precious time of medical staff); anger and frustration (about time wasted, about not being taken seriously, about not being treated quickly enough); doubt (about the reality of pain—what if it's all in my head?). And faced with the challenge of communicating pain, the sufferer may find that none of her expressions—linguistic or bodily—applies.

There is, and shall remain, an asymmetry of knowledge about what is happening to a person who is in pain. Those with expert knowledge will always know more about what is happening to the body and brain of that person. But the person who is comprised of that body and brain will always know better how it feels to be himself, in pain. Experience and epistemology do not, as things are, readily converge. Since the meaningfulness of pain is created in the brain via a combination of neuroscientific, biological constants, and the context and experience of the individual sufferer, what pain *means* and how pain *feels* will always be liable to variation. Pain experience will vary even in the same individual. The possibilities for the potential for variance across time, place, and culture are striking. The alleviation of pain—and often this will mean that the focus must shift from *diagnosis* to *management*, especially in cases of chronic pain—may involve the medical establishment becoming more literate in the language of pain of their patients. There would have to be a conscious understanding of the way in which the available expressions of pain—verbal, gestural, postural, artistic, stoic, etc.—are factored into a thorough appraisal of pain experience. One first step towards this openness to cultures of pain would be to relinquish the quest to define pain.

References

Chapter 1: Pain concepts

Al-Jeilani, Mohamed, 'Pain: Points of View of Islamic Theology', *Acta Neurochirurgica Suppl*, 38 (1987): 132–5.

Maalej, Zouhair, 'Figurative Language in Anger Expressions in Tunisian Arabic: An Extended View of Embodiment', *Metaphor and Symbol*, 19 (2004): 51–75.

Merskey, H., 'Some Features of the History of the Idea of Pain', *Pain*, 9 (1980): 3–8.

Santangelo, Paolo, 'The Perception of Pain in Late-Imperial China', in Rob Boddice (ed.), *Pain and Emotion in Modern History* (Houndmills: Palgrave, 2014).

Tu, Wei-Ming, 'A Chinese Perspective on Pain', *Acta Neurochirurgica Suppl.*, 38 (1987): 147–51.

Chapter 2: Pain and piety

Chen, Lih-Mik, C. Miaskowski, M. Dodd, and S. Pantilat, 'Concepts within the Chinese Culture that Influence the Cancer Pain Experience', *Cancer Nursing*, 31 (2008): 103–8.

Moscoso, Javier, *Pain: A Cultural History* (Basingstoke: Palgrave, 2012).

Chapter 3: Pain and the machine

Harrison, A., 'Arabic Pain Words', *Pain*, 32 (1988): 239–50.

Costa, Luciola da Cunha Menezes, Christopher G. Maher, James H. McAuley, and Leonardo Oliveira Pena Costa, 'Systematic Review of

Cross-cultural Adaptations of McGill Pain Questionnaire Reveals a
Paucity of Clinimetric Testing', *Journal of Clinical Epidemiology*,
62 (2009): 934–43.

Chapter 4: Pain and civilization

Eastman, Peggy, 'Genetic and Ethnic Differences Reported in Pain
Perception', *Neurology Today*, 9 (2009): 20–2.

Miller, Carly, and Sarah E. Newton, 'Pain Perception and Expression:
The Influence of Gender, Personal Self-Efficacy, and Lifespan
Socialization', *Pain Management Nursing*, 7 (2006): 148–52
(quoting M. McCaffrey).

Page, Gayle Giboney, 'Are There Long-Term Consequences of Pain in
Newborn or Very Young Infants?', *Journal of Perinatal Education*,
13 (2004): 10–17.

Schiavenato, M., J.F. Byers, P. Scovanner, J.M. McMahon, Y. Xia, N. Lu,
and H. He, 'Neonatal Pain Facial Expression: Evaluating the Primal
Face of Pain', *Pain*, 138 (2008): 460–71.

Wood, Whitney, '"When I Think of What is Before Me, I Feel Afraid":
Narratives of Fear, Pain and Childbirth in Late Victorian Canada',
in Rob Boddice (ed.), *Pain and Emotion in Modern History*
(Houndmills: Palgrave, 2014): 187–203.

Woodrow, Kenneth, Gary Friedman, A.B. Siegelaub, and Morris F.
Collen, 'Pain Tolerance: Differences According to Age, Sex and Race',
Psychosomatic Medicine, 34 (1972): 548–56.

Zatzick, D.F., and J.E. Dimsdale, 'Cultural Variations in Response to
Painful Stimuli', *Psychosomatic Medicine*, 52 (1990).

Chapter 5: Sympathy, compassion, empathy

Haskell, Thomas, 'Capitalism and the Origins of Humanitarian
Sensibility, Part 1', *American Historical Review*, 90 (1985): 339–61.

Chapter 6: Pain as pleasure

Berbara, Maria, '"Esta Pena Tan Sabrosa": Teresa of Avila and the
Figurative Arts', in Jan Frans van Dijkhuizen and Karl A.E.
Enenkel (eds), *The Sense of Suffering: Constructions of Physical
Pain in Early Modern Culture* (Leiden: Brill, 2009): 267–97.

Ellis, Havelock, 'Love and Pain', *Studies in the Psychology of Sex*, vol. 3
(Philadelphia: F.A. Davis and Co., 1920): 66–188.

Mieszkowski, Jan, 'Fear of a Safe Place', in Jan Plamper and Benjamin Lazier (eds), *Fear Across the Disciplines* (Pittsburgh: University of Pittsburgh Press, 2012): 99–117.

Chapter 7: Pain in modern medicine and science

Fields, Howard L., 'Setting the Stage for Pain: Allegorical Tales from Neuroscience', in Sarah Coakley and Kay Kaufman Shelemay (eds), *Pain and Its Transformations: The Interface of Biology and Culture* (Cambridge, MA: Harvard University Press, 2007): 36–61.

Hall, K.T., J. Loscalzo, and T.J. Kaptchuk, 'Genetics and the Placebo Effect: The Placebome', *Trends in Molecular Medicine*, 21 (2015): 285–94.

Kugelmann, Robert, 'Pain in the Vernacular: Psychological and Physical', *Journal of Health Psychology*, 5 (2000): 305–13.

Melzack, Ronald, and Patrick Wall, 'Pain Mechanisms: A New Theory', *Science*, n.s. 150 (1965): 971–9.

Tuttle, Alexander, Sarasa Tohyama, Tim Ramsay, Jonathan Kimmelman, Petra Schweinhardt, Gary Bennett, and Jeffrey Mogil, 'Increasing Placebo Responses Over Time in U.S. Clinical Trials of Neuropathic Pain', *Pain*, 156 (2015).

Chapter 8: Chronic pain

Campbell, Gabrielle, Shane Darke, Raimondo Bruno, and Louisa Degenhardt, 'The Prevalence and Correlates of Chronic Pain and Suicidality in a Nationally Representative Sample', *Australian and New Zealand Journal of Psychiatry*, 49 (2015): 803–11.

Goldberg, Daniel, *The Bioethics of Pain Management: Beyond Opioids* (New York: Routledge, 2014).

Harstall, Christa, 'How Prevalent Is Chronic Pain?', *Pain Clinical Updates*, 11 (2003): 1–4.

Melzack, Ronald, 'Evolution of the Neuromatrix Theory of Pain', *Pain Practice*, 5 (2005): 85–94.

Torrance, Nicola, Alison M. Elliott, Amanda J. Lee, and Blair H. Smith, 'Severe Chronic Pain is Associated with Increased 10 Year Mortality: A Cohort Record Linkage Study', *European Journal of Pain*, 14 (2010): 380–6.

Vaso, Apostol, Haim-Moshe Adahan, Artan Gjika, Skerdi Zahaj, Tefik Zhurda, Gentian Vyshka, and Marshall Devor, 'Peripheral Nervous System Origin of Phantom Limb Pain', *Pain*, 155 (2014): 1384–91.

Zeidan, F., J.A. Grant, C.A. Brown, J.G. McHaffie, and R.C. Coghill, 'Mindfulness Meditation-related Pain Relief: Evidence for Unique Brain Mechanisms in the Regulation of Pain', *Neuroscience Letters*, 520 (2012): 165–73.

Chapter 9: Cultures of pain

Gellar, Pamela L., 'Altering Identities: Body Modifications and the Pre-Columbian Maya', in Christopher Knüsel and Rebecca Gowland (eds), *Social Archaeology of Funerary Remains* (Oxford: Oxford University Press, 2009).

Padfield, Deborah, 'Mirrors in the Darkness: Pain and Photography, Natural Partners', *Qualia*, 1 (2016).

Further reading

History of pain

Bending, Lucy, *The Representation of Bodily Pain in Nineteenth-century English Culture* (Oxford: Oxford University Press, 2000).

Boddice, Rob, ed., *Pain and Emotion in Modern History* (Basingstoke: Palgrave, 2014).

Bourke, Joanna, *The Story of Pain: From Prayer to Painkillers* (Oxford: Oxford University Press, 2014).

Bourke, Joanna, Louise Hide, and Carmen Mangion, eds, 'Perspectives on Pain', *19: Interdisciplinary Studies in the Long Nineteenth Century*, 15 (2012).

Cohen, Esther, *The Modulated Scream: Pain in Late Medieval Culture* (Chicago: University of Chicago Press, 2010).

Cohen, Esther, Leona Toker, Manuela Consonni, and Otniel Dror, eds, *Knowledge and Pain* (Amsterdam: Rodopi, 2012).

Dijkhuizen, Jan Frans van, *Pain and Compassion in Early Modern English Literature and Culture* (Cambridge: D.S. Brewer, 2012).

Dijkhuizen, Jan Frans van, and Karl A.E. Enenkel, eds, *The Sense of Suffering: Constructions of Physical Pain in Early Modern Culture* (Leiden and Boston: Brill, 2009).

Dormandy, Thomas, *The Worst of Evils: The Fight Against Pain* (New Haven: Yale University Press, 2006).

Hodgkiss, Andrew, *From Lesion to Metaphor: Chronic Pain in British, French and German Medical Writings, 1800–1914* (Amsterdam: Rodopi, 2000).

Jackson, S.W., *Care of the Psyche: A History of Psychological Healing* (New Haven: Yale University Press, 1999).

Mann, Ronald D., *The History of the Management of Pain: From Early Principles to Present Practice* (Carnforth: Parthenon Publishing, 1988).

Merback, M.B., *The Thief, the Cross and the Wheel: Pain and the Spectacle of Punishment in Medieval and Renaissance Europe* (Chicago: Chicago University Press, 1999).

Merskey, H., 'Some Features of the History of the Idea of Pain', *Pain*, 9 (1980): 3–8.

Mills, Robert, ed., *Suspended Animation: Pain, Pleasure and Punishment in Medieval Culture* (London: Reaktion, 2006).

Morris, David B., *The Culture of Pain* (Berkeley: University of California Press, 1991).

Moscoso, Javier, *Pain: A Cultural History* (Basingstoke: Palgrave, 2012).

Perkins, Judith, *The Suffering Self: Pain and Narrative Representation in the Early Christian Era* (London: Routledge, 1995).

Pernick, Martin S., *A Calculus of Suffering: Pain, Professionalism, and Anesthesia in Nineteenth-century America* (New York: Columbia University Press, 1985).

Price, Douglas B., and Neil J. Twombly, *The Phantom Limb Phenomenon: A Medical, Folkloric, and Historical Study: Texts and Translations of 10th to 20th Century Accounts of the Miraculous Restoration of Lost Body Parts* (Washington, DC: Georgetown University Press, 1978).

Rey, Roselyne, *The History of Pain* (Cambridge, MA: Harvard University Press, 1998).

Van Dijkhuizen, Jan Frans, and Karl A.E. Enenkel, *The Sense of Suffering: Constructions of Physical Pain in Early Modern Culture* (Leiden: Brill, 2009).

Vertosick, Frank T., *Why We Hurt: The Natural History of Pain* (New York: Harcourt, 2000).

Yamamoto-Wilson, John R., *Pain, Pleasure and Perversity: Discourses of Suffering in Seventeenth-century England* (Farnham: Ashgate, 2013).

Contemporary pain medicine and science

Baszanger, Isabelle, *Inventing Pain Medicine: From the Laboratory to the Clinic* (New Brunswick, NJ: Rutgers University Press, 1998).

Biro, David, *The Language of Pain: Finding Words, Compassion, and Relief* (New York: Norton, 2000).

Chapman, C. Richard, 'A Passion of the Soul: An Introduction to Pain for Consciousness Researchers', *Consciousness and Cognition*, 8 (1999): 391–422.

Fields, Howard L., 'Setting the Stage for Pain: Allegorical Tales from Neuroscience', in Sarah Coakley and Kay Kaufman Shelemay (eds), *Pain and Its Transformations: The Interface of Biology and Culture* (Cambridge, MA: Harvard University Press, 2007): 36–61.

Foreman, Judy, *A Nation in Pain: Healing Our Biggest Health Problem* (New York: Oxford University Press, 2014).

Gatchel, Robert J., Yuan Bo Peng, Madelon L. Peters, Perry N. Fuchs, and Dennis C. Turk, 'The Biopsychosocial Approach to Chronic Pain: Scientific Advances and Future Directions', *Psychological Bulletin*, 133 (2007): 581–624.

Grahek, Nikola, *Feeling Pain and Being in Pain* (2nd edn., Cambridge, MA: MIT Press, 2007).

Kugelmann, Robert, 'Pain in the Vernacular: Psychological and Physical', *Journal of Health Pscyhology*, 5 (2000): 305–13.

Livingston, William K., *Pain and Suffering* (Seattle: IASP Press, 1998).

MacDonald, Geoff, and Lauri A. Jensen-Campbell, eds, *Social Pain: Neuropsychological and Health Implications of Loss and Exclusion* (Washington, DC: American Psychological Association, 2011).

Melzack, R., 'Evolution of the Neuromatrix Theory of Pain', *Pain Practice*, 5 (2005): 85–94.

Melzack, R., and P.D. Wall, *The Challenge of Pain* (London: Penguin, 1996).

Merskey, H., 'International Association for the Study of Pain: Classification of Chronic Pain: Descriptions of Chronic Pain Syndromes and Definitions of Pain Terms', *Pain*, 3 (1986): 1–226.

Wall, Patrick, *Pain: The Science of Suffering* (New York: Columbia University Press, 2002).

Anaesthesia and pain killers

Bankoff, George, *The Conquest of Pain: The Story of Anaesthesia* (London: Macdonald & Co., 1940).

Canton, Donald, *What a Blessing She Had Chloroform: The Medical and Social Response to the Pain of Childbirth from 1800 to the Present* (New Haven: Yale University Press, 1999).

Ellis, E.S., *Ancient Anodynes: Primitive Anaesthesia and Allied Conditions* (London: Heinemann, 1946).

Fülöp-Miller, René, *Triumph over Pain* (Indianapolis: Bobbs-Merrill, 1938).

Pöll, Johan Sebastian, *The Anaesthetist, 1890–1960: A Historical Comparative Study between Britain and Germany* (Rotterdam: Erasmus, 2011).

McTavish, Jan R., *Pain & Profits: The History of the Headache and Its Remedies in America* (New Brunswick, NJ: Rutgers University Press, 2004).

Snow, Stephanie J., *Operations Without Pain: The Practice and Science of Anaesthesia in Victorian Britain* (Basingstoke: Palgrave, 2006).

Social and political studies

Folkmarson Käll, Lisa, *Dimensions of Pain: Humanities and Social Science Perspectives* (London: Routledge, 2013).

Goldberg, Daniel, *The Bioethics of Pain Management: Beyond Opioids* (New York: Routledge, 2014).

Lewis, C.S., *The Problem of Pain* (1940; New York: Harper Collins, 2001).

Scarry, Elaine, *The Body in Pain* (Oxford: Oxford University Press, 1987).

Sontag, Susan, *Regarding the Pain of Others* (New York: Picador, 2003).

Wailoo, Keith, *Pain: A Political History* (Baltimore: Johns Hopkins University Press, 2014).

Art and literature

Berry, Michael, *A History of Pain: Trauma in Modern Chinese Literature and Film* (New York: Columbia University Press, 2008).

Davies, Jeremy, *Bodily Pain in Romantic Literature* (New York: Routledge, 2014).

Di Bella, Maria Pia, and James Elkins, eds, *Representations of Pain in Art and Visual Culture* (New York: Routledge, 2013).

Mintz, Susannah B., *Hurt and Pain: Literature and the Suffering Body* (London: Bloomsbury, 2013).

Norridge, Zoe, *Perceiving Pain in African Literature* (Houndmills: Palgrave, 2013).

Padfield, Deborah, *Perceptions of Pain* (Stockport: Dewi Lewis, 2003).

Pascual, Nieves, ed., *Witness to Pain: Essays on the Translation of Pain into Art* (Bern: Peter Lang, 2005).

Spivey, Nigel, *Enduring Creation: Art, Pain, and Fortitude* (Berkeley: University of California Press, 2001).

Index

A

A delta fibres 82
acetaminophen 63–4, 90–2
Achilles 6
acupuncture 12, 112
addiction 117
adrenaline 83, 92
affect 7, 39–42, 44, 72, 76, 80, 82,
    86–91, 100, 102, 108
African Americans 49
Al-Jeilani, Mohamed 13
'alam 13
algometer 36
algos 6–7
allodynia 82
American Civil War 98
anaesthesia 5, 25, 32–3, 54–5,
    79–80, 82, 87, 112
analgesics 13–14, 35, 45, 90–1, 93
anandamide 92
ancient Greece 6–9, 57
anger 10, 13, 47, 75, 103–4, 118
anguish 3, 6–7, 9, 12–13, 18, 54,
    112, 115
animal pain 27–8, 30–4, 46, 49,
    62, 65
anti-depressants 103
anxiety 12, 43, 47, 54–6, 72, 83, 86,
    90, 103–4, 110

Arabic 13, 41
Aristotle (384–322 BCE) 7, 10, 60
art 15, 68, 70, 73, 108, 113–16
asceticism 16, 20, 24, 65
aspirin 90–1
Aurelius, Marcus (121–80 CE) 94
    Meditations 94

B

babies 46–7
back pain 1, 95
Bacon, Francis (1909–92) 114–16
    Three Studies for a
        Crucifixion 114–15
Beecher, Henry (1904–76) 85, 99
behaviourism 34–5, 39
Bell, Charles (1774–1842) 109–10
Bentham, Jeremy (1748–1832) 30–1
Berbara, Maria 68
Bernini, Gian Lorenzo 68
    Ecstasy of Saint Teresa 68
biology 12, 49, 78
biopsychosocial model 2, 93, 111
Bois-Reymond, Emil du (1818–96)
    36
Bonica, John (1917–94) 1, 112
Bourke, Joanna 45
brain 3, 37–8, 46, 53, 59–61, 66, 72,
    78–91, 98–101, 104, 106–8, 118

Breule, Gualterus 11
broken heart 63, 90
Buddhism 24
Burke, Edmund (1729–97)
    57, 67
    *Philosophical Enquiry into the
    Origin of Our Ideas of the
    Sublime and Beautiful* 67
burning 7, 81, 84, 94, 97, 101
Burton, Robert (1577–1640) 10
    Anatomy of Melancholy 10

C

C fibres 82
cannabinoids 92
capsaicin 81
Catholicism 18, 23, 30, 43,
    69, 73
ch'i (qi) 12
Charcot, Jean-Martin (1825–93) 51,
    110–11
Chen, Lih-Mik 24
Chidi Mari 106
childbirth 17, 20, 32–3, 45–9
childhood 45–6
China 12, 24, 112
chloroform 32, 55, 79
Crichton-Browne, James
    (1840–1938) 32
Christ 7–8, 15–19, 23–4,
    114, 116
Christianity 15–20, 22, 24, 26,
    30, 116
chronic pain 1–2, 41–2, 79–80, 82,
    84, 93, 94–104 *passim* 108,
    113, 118
Cohen, Esther 11, 20
communication 3, 12, 34, 96, 102,
    106, 111, 114, 118
compassion 17, 35–6, 52–4, 57, 63,
    67, 95
Confucianism 12, 24
congenital analgesia 65, 86–7
cortisol 102–4

crucifixion 15, 19, 114, 115
cruelty 25, 62, 74–5
cyberball 90

D

dard 12–13
Darwin, Charles (1809–82) 25,
    33–4, 56–9
    Descent of Man 57
    On the Origin of Species 58
Daston, Lorraine 39
David, Gerard (1460–1523) 21–2
    Judgement of Cambyses 22
death 5, 8, 19–20, 31, 67, 69, 73,
    94, 113–14, 115
definition 1–2, 11, 14, 44, 56, 60,
    77, 88, 91, 95–6, 102, 113, 118
Descartes, René (1596–1650) 14,
    27–32, 37, 98
    Discourse on Method 30
    Meditations 28
    Treatise on Man 28–9
Devor, Marshall 101
Dimsdale, J.E. 49
Diogenes Laertius (3rd century
    CE) 9
discipline 20, 24–5, 69, 73, 75
disease 10, 20, 32, 35, 50, 52, 78,
    96–7, 111
disgust 61, 66–7
dolor 9
dolore 9, 17
dolorimeter *see* algometer
dopamine 91–2
douleur 9
dualism 6, 12, 14, 27, 29, 35, 77,
    79, 95, 100, 117
duhkh 13

E

Ecce Homo 15
ecstasy 68–9, 72
effeminacy 50

Pain

Eisenberger, Naomi 90
eleos 57
Ellis, Havelock (1859–1939) 74–5
emotional control 50, 103
emotional pain 2, 12, 23, 51, 56, 58, 63–4, 77, 79, 88, 90–1, 110–11
empathy 3–4, 53, 59–64
endogenous opioids 3, 60, 91–2
endorphins 91
Enlightenment 22, 27, 31, 46, 54
epinephrine *see* adrenaline
Erichsen, John Eric (1818–96) 51
Eros 69, 73
ether 32, 55
evolution 17, 34, 49, 56–7, 59, 65, 74–5, 87, 97
expression 34, 41, 45–6, 61, 68, 96, 106–7, 109–10, 112–16, 118

F

Fanny Hill 70
fear 7, 9, 30–1, 47–8, 55–6, 61, 67, 72, 75, 83, 85–6, 90–1, 104, 106–7, 118
Fields, Howard 84
First World War 33, 52, 94, 99
flagellation 20, 24, 73, 75
Flood, Gavin 24
Foreman, Judy 78
Freud, Sigmund (1856–1939) 67
functional magnetic resonance imaging (fMRI) 3, 59, 63, 87–8, 104, 108

G

Galen of Pergamon (129–200/216 CE) 9–11
Galison, Peter 39
gate control theory 79–82, 84–5, 99, 112
Gellar, Pamela 107
gender 35–6, 38, 44–5, 50, 52, 106, 114, 117

Genesis 17, 94
genetics 49, 63, 87, 92, 100–1, 104
God 13, 18, 20–1, 23–6, 68
Goldberg, Daniel 96
Golden Rule 58
grief 3, 6–7, 9–11, 13, 15, 16–17, 90–1, 115
gun-shot wound 79

H

Harrison, Ann 41
Harvard Medical School 92
Haskell, Thomas 62–3
headache 1, 11, 52, 91
Hercules (Heracles) 7, 8
Hinduism 24, 106
Hogarth, William 70
   Harlot's Progress 70
Holy Roman Empire 18
homeostasis 78
Homer 6
   Iliad 7
humanity 17, 19, 25, 31, 44, 62, 66–7
Hume, David (1711–76) 54, 57
humorism 9–11
hurt 2, 6–7, 15, 23, 58, 78–9, 85, 90, 96, 106, 117
hyperalgesia 82
hypnotism 112
hysteria 50, 99, 108–11

I

Ichneumon wasp 25
illness 10, 23, 46, 50–2, 66, 98–9, 104, 117
imitatio Christi 18
immune system 83, 102
India 12
injury 2, 7, 11–12, 15, 28–9, 32, 35, 38, 40, 46, 51, 58, 60, 63–5, 67, 72, 77–8, 80–91 *passim* 95–7, 99–102, 104, 108, 115

Index

International Association for the
    Study of Pain (IASP) 1, 11,
    77, 96

J

James, E.L. (b. 1963) 75
    Fifty Shades of Grey 75
Jews 49
justice 17, 21
Justinian (483–565 CE) 8

K

Kama Sutra 72–3
Kinbaku 73 *see also* Shibari
Konstan, David 57
Koran 13
Krafft Ebing, Richard von
    (1840–1902) 70
Kugelmann, Robert 77
Kuhn, Thomas (1922–96) 39

L

labour (parturition) 17, 32–3
labour (work) 17, 94
Latin 7, 9–10, 14, 17, 57, 70, 78
Latour, Bruno (b. 1947) 39
Leid 9
lesion 2, 28, 51, 82, 86, 88, 95, 98
Lewis, C.S. (1898–1963) 25–6
lobotomy 88
Lombroso, Cesare 36
    Criminal Man 36
love 6, 24–6, 66, 68, 70, 73–4
lupé 7

M

Maalej, Zouhair 13
McGill Pain Questionnaire 40–2
Man of Sorrows 15–16, 116
Mard 13

Marshall, Henry Rutgers
    (1852–1927) 39
martyrs 17, 20–4, 26, 65, 73
masochism 69, 73–4
Maurus of Salerno (1130–1214) 11
measurement 2, 34–5, 39, 105
mechanisms 26–34 *passim* 37–40,
    53, 59–60, 63–4, 81, 82, 112,
    117
Meibom, Heinrich (1590–1655)
    70, 72
melancholy 10, 50
Melzack, Ronald (b. 1929) 40,
    80–1, 99–101, 106, 117
mercy 57
Merskey, Harold 11
metaphor 4, 6, 37, 39–40, 53, 94,
    96, 113
Mieszkowski, Jan 67
Mill, John Stuart (1806–73) 58
    On Liberty 58
Miller, Carly 45
mindfulness 103
mirror neurons 61
misericordia 57
Mitchell, Silas Weir (1829–1914) 98
Mogil, Jeffrey 92
morality 12, 17, 30–1, 35, 43, 58–9,
    62–3, 66, 70, 98, 111
Morgan, Conwy Lloyd (1852–1936)
    34, 39
Morgan's canon 39
Morris, David B. (b. 1942) 86
Morton, William T.G. (1819–68) 32
Moscoso, Javier 16
multiple sclerosis 94

N

narcotics 45, 117
needles 56, 85
neo-utilitarianism 65
nerves 3, 38, 43, 50, 52, 55, 78, 80,
    82, 99

Pain

nervous system 38, 46–7, 51, 78, 82–4, 92, 97–8, 101, 106–7
neurasthenia 43, 52
neuroimaging 59, 66, 87, 107
neuromatrix 99–101
neuroplasticity 99–100, 102, 104, 107
neuroscience 3, 38–9, 53, 60–1, 63, 88, 90, 102, 107, 118
Newton, Sarah 45
Nietzsche, Friedrich (1844–1900) 113–14, 115
nociception 38, 77–80, 82

O

objectivity 33, 35, 39, 41
odune 7
oiktos 57
opioids 3, 64, 66, 91, 117
Osler, William (1849–1919) 55
oxytocin 91

P

Padfield, Deborah 113
Page, Gale 47
pain asymbolia *see* congenital analgesia
pain killers *see* analgesics
pain management 1–2, 5, 13, 39, 50, 80, 102, 104, 108, 111, 116, 118
pain pathway 28, 29, 37, 79–80, 82
pain syndromes 40, 42, 93, 104, 110
paracetamol *see* acetaminophen
Paré, Ambroise (1510–90) 98
passions 6–7, 9–10, 15–17, 114
patience 13, 23
pattern theories 38–9, 80
phantom pain 39, 98–102
pharmaceuticals 92–3
phenomenology 14, 100

Pieta 17
piety 16–17, 22
pity 9, 17, 54, 57, 60, 67–8
placebo 91–3, 112
Plato 56, 66–7
  Republic 67
pleasure 30–1, 39, 43, 48, 54, 58, 66–76 *passim*
Plutarch (45–120 CE) 30
politics 14, 41, 44, 50, 53, 57, 106
post-traumatic stress 51, 99
Protestantism 24, 69
Providence 20
psychogenic pain 99, 117
psychology 34, 36–7, 39, 46, 52, 63, 74, 77, 96, 98–100
punishment 14–15, 17–18, 20–2, 83–4

R

race 35–6, 48–9, 62
railway spine 51–2
real-time fMRI 104, 108
reflex 28, 32, 34, 65, 83
Reformation 16, 18, 24, 69
rites of passage 106
ritual 74, 106–7
runner's high 66
Ryder, Richard (b. 194) 65

S

Sacher-Masoch, Leopold von 73
  Venus im Pelz 73–4
Sade, Marquis de 70
sadism 70–3
Sanskrit 13
Santangelo, Paolo 12
Scarry, Elaine 96, 106
  The Body in Pain 106
Schadenfreude 66
Scheler, Max (1874–1928) 56
Schiavenato, Martin 46

Index

Schmerz 9

Schmerzensmann *see* Man of Sorrows

Schrenck-Notzing, Albert von (1862–1929) 74

sciatica 94

Scott, Joan (b. 1941) 114

Second World War 25, 99

self-pity 68

Seneca 10

sensibility *see* sensitivity

sensitivity 3, 25, 35–7, 43–4, 46–7, 49, 64, 69, 81–2, 98, 117

sentience 12, 46

serotonin 91–2

sex 69–76 *passim* 98, 111

Shadwell, Thomas 70

Shibari 73

shingles 104

Simpson, James Young (1811–70) 32

sin 18–20, 23–5

Sint Jans, Geergten tot 15–16

Man of Sorrows 15, 16

slavery 57, 62–3, 73–4

Smith, Adam (1723–90) 56–8

social pain 63, 88, 89, 90, 103

soldiers 79, 85–6, 99–100

Sontag, Susan (1933–2004) 54, 66

Regarding the Pain of Others 66

sorrow 9, 11, 13, 15, 17, 116

soul 6, 9, 18, 20, 24, 27–8, 30–1, 46, 68

Spencer, Herbert (1820–1903) 67

Stilinović, Mladen (b. 1947) 113

Stoicism 8–10, 24, 94

stress 47, 102–4

suffering 2–3, 6–13, 15–20, 23–6, 28–31, 33, 35, 37, 43, 47, 52, 54, 57–60, 62–4, 66–7, 69, 74, 91, 95–7, 99, 102–7, 110, 113–16, 118

suicide 74, 95

surgery 32, 46, 54–5, 79, 93, 98

Susini, Clemente (1754–1814) 68

sympathy 3, 47, 53–9, 63, 67

T

Tagore, Rabrindranath (1861–1941) 13

Taoism 12

Teresa of Ávila 68

terror 48, 54–5, 67

tetanus 109–11

theology 15, 18–21, 24–6, 69

theory of mind 59–61

threat 60, 86, 97

Torgeson, Warren (1924–99) 40

torture 12, 15, 17, 20–2, 25, 106

translation 17, 40–2, 61

Tu, Wei-Ming 12

Tylenol 92

U

University College Hospital 113

Utilitarianism 26, 30–1, 43, 58, 65

V

vaccination 55–6, 111

van Dijkhuizen, Jan Frans 11

Venere dei Medici 68

vir dolorum *see* Man of Sorrows

vivisection (animal experimentation) 31–4

W

Wall, Patrick (1925–2001) 28, 77, 80–1, 85–6, 99, 106, 112, 117

witches 19

women 32, 44–5, 47–9, 52, 74, 111–12

Woodrow, Kenneth 49

World Health Organization (WHO) 55–6

wounds 4, 6, 15–16, 18, 40, 79, 87

Y

Yamamoto-Wilson, John 69
Yom Kippur War 99

Z

Zatzick, D.F. 49
Zedong, Mao (1893–1976) 112

Index

SOCIAL MEDIA
Very Short Introduction

Join our community
www.oup.com/vsi

- Join us online at the official Very Short Introductions **Facebook** page.
- Access the thoughts and musings of our authors with our online **blog**.
- Sign up for our monthly **e-newsletter** to receive information on all new titles publishing that month.
- Browse the full range of Very Short Introductions online.
- Read **extracts** from the Introductions for free.
- If you are a teacher or lecturer you can order inspection copies quickly and simply via our website.